Praise for

SEASONAL
SELF-CARE
RITUALS

"This book is a must for anyone who wants to understand how to stay healthy throughout the year. Drawing on her extensive training, as well as decades of personal experience, Susan Weis-Bohlen takes the teachings of Ayurvedic seasonal routines and makes them accessible to all, providing us with a wide variety of practices to stay balanced and healthy in body, mind, and spirit. Complete with recipes and simple practices, *Seasonal Self-Care Rituals* is an invaluable resource for improving our overall well-being."

—*Sheila Patel, MD, chief medical officer for Chopra Global*

"This gem of a book is like having a personal mind-body coach. Susan is a masterful teacher whose rituals, delicious recipes, and transformational practices keep us in thrive mode every day by aligning with nature. I will drink in the riches of this treasure for many years to come!"

—*davidji, author of* Sacred Powers

"*Seasonal Self-Care Rituals* is an excellent guide to understanding the cycles of nature and how our physiology responds to various seasons of life. This is the true essence of personalized medicine. "

—*Dr. Suhas Kshirsagar BAMS, MD, author of* Change Your Schedule, Change Your Life *and* The Hot Belly Diet

"If you want to play and work more skillfully with your health, your doshas, and the seasons, this is the book for you. Susan Weis-Bohlen is the ultimate Ayurvedic woman next door: supportive, informative, clear, nurturing, and down to earth. Susan, conscious of the interface of belief, feeling, and biology, tends your curious mind as well as your tender heart. Appealing, accessible, affordable, with delicious recipes—what more could you want?"

—*Amadea Morningstar, Ayurveda educator and author of* Easy Healing Drinks from the Wisdom of Ayurveda *and* Ayurvedic Cooking for Westerners

"Books about the ancient system of Ayurveda can be cumbersome and confusing—but not Susan's! Every word is beautiful and rich; forever, will I use Susan's book to make natural choices that are as simple as 'flowing downstream.'"

—*Cyndi Dale, intuitive, healer, and author twenty-six books, including* Energy Healing for Trauma, Stress & Chronic Illness

"*Seasonal Self-Care Rituals* is a comprehensive yet welcoming entree to how to use Ayurveda's wisdom and practice self-care according to constitution and climate. Readers are sure to benefit."

—*Kate O'Donnell, author of* The Everyday Ayurveda Cookbook, Everyday Ayurveda Cooking for a Calm, Clear Mind, *and* The Everyday Ayurveda Guide to Self-Care

"This book is my go-to resource for natural health! The practicality, applicability, accessibility of Susan's work stands out—and she masterfully weaves healing routines with a sensory and spiritual experience, leading us in its application literally step-by-step. This book is a treasure!"

—*Amanda Ree, founder of Sama Dog Wellbeing and a Chopra-certified Ayurveda, meditation, and yoga instructor*

"*Seasonal Self-Care Rituals* validates Nobel Prize–winning circadian science with the ancient and practical wisdom of Ayurveda's seasonal life cycles."

—*Dr. John Douillard DC, CAP founder of LifeSpa.com*

"*Seasonal Self-Care Rituals* focuses on how we can integrate Ayurveda into our lives to experience well-being according to our own personal natures. This book will help readers to pay attention to Mother Nature, working with her to make informed life choices. The more we learn about ourselves, the better we can follow our own individual paths to nurturance, health, and true satisfaction in life."

—*Dr. Robert Svoboda, Ayurvedic physician and author of* Prakriti: Your Ayurvedic Constitution

"*Seasonal Self-Care Rituals* takes you to the roots and rhythms of Ayurveda, through the different seasons. Susan is your guide to eat, breathe, move, and sleep better. This is a book that will guide you through baby steps, inspire you for profound changes, and make you flow in harmony with nature through the stages of life!"

—*Ramkumar Kutty, BAMS, founder and director of Punarnava Ayurveda*

SEASONAL SELF-CARE RITUALS

EAT, BREATHE, MOVE, AND SLEEP BETTER— ACCORDING TO YOUR DOSHA

SUSAN WEIS-BOHLEN

TILLER PRESS

New York   London   Toronto   Sydney   New Delhi

TILLER PRESS

An Imprint of Simon & Schuster, Inc.
1230 Avenue of the Americas
New York, NY 10020

First Tiller Press hardcover edition December 2020

TILLER PRESS and colophon are trademarks of Simon & Schuster, Inc.

For information about special discounts for bulk purchases, please contact Simon & Schuster Special Sales at 1-866-506-1949 or business@simonandschuster.com.

The Simon & Schuster Speakers Bureau can bring authors to your live event. For more information or to book an event, contact the Simon & Schuster Speakers Bureau at 1-866-248-3049 or visit our website at www.simonspeakers.com.

Interior design by Jennifer Chung

Manufactured in the United States of America

1 3 5 7 9 10 8 6 4 2

Library of Congress Cataloging-in-Publication Data has been applied for.

ISBN 978-1-9821-5218-5
ISBN 978-1-9821-5220-8 (ebook)

To all the mothers who have loved
and supported me unconditionally . . .

my mom, Bunny,
my mother-in-law, Mary Lou,
and Mother Nature

CONTENTS

INTRODUCTION

When I was twenty-nine years old, long before bookstores had chairs and cozy reading corners or I owned my own bookshop, and years before I had even heard the word "Ayurveda," I found myself sitting on the floor of Crown Books in Washington, DC. I had come across a book called *Ageless Body, Timeless Mind: The Quantum Alternative to Growing Old* by a young Indian doctor named Deepak Chopra. The flap of the book had a quote by Wayne Dyer: "Who might have imagined that the secret to conquering this universal mystery [of aging] lies not in our physical bodies but in our consciousness?" The introduction went on to say, "By intervening at the level where belief becomes biology, we can achieve our unbound potential." I learned while flipping through the pages that if one is feeling sad, it's not just in the brain, but all over the body—"belief becomes biology." We can use our own abilities to create our reality. Our internal dialogue is just random mental noise coming from beliefs and assumptions—and this was just up to page 26!

I was hooked. This was 1993 and bookstores didn't encourage reading in the stacks in those days, but that didn't stop me from making myself at home and devouring much of the book on the spot. *Ageless Body, Timeless Mind* was the key to discovering who I truly was. Although Ayurveda isn't even mentioned in this book until page 269, that first exploration of a consciousness-based lifestyle that relies on food, yoga, meditation, and seasonal rituals to harmonize and heal the mind, body, and soul captured my attention and never let go.

I bought the book and took it back to my apartment, and my consciousness began a slow and subtle shift. At the time I was newly arrived in Washington, DC, after nearly a decade living in Israel. I had a fascinating job at the Israeli embassy, lived a tiny but cute apartment, and was dating a lot of guys. But I was depressed, overweight, and bulimic. I was seeing a therapist and going to Weight Watchers, but was still a mess.

Reading this book, I saw for the first time that mind and body were connected. The ancient Indian wisdom Chopra wrote about fascinated me, its messages subtle yet unmistakable: If we eat right, live a peaceful lifestyle, and practice meditation and yoga, we can begin to hear the messages coming from within. *You are already perfect. You have all the answers. Only you know your path. Just be still and listen.*

My own path led me to explore meditation, which in turn taught me deep self-acceptance and faith in my intuition. All at once I felt I had been given permission: *I don't have to be what everyone thinks I should be! I can forge my own path! Finally!*

With this deep knowing in my back pocket, nearly 10 years later, in 2002, while in L.A. attending a PR/marketing conference for the Baltimore-based company I worked for, I walked into the fabled Bodhi Tree bookstore. As I made my way through the stacks, a feeling washed over me that I needed to open a bookstore just like this, offering metaphysical books, classes, talks, and workshops. The Chopra book (and several more of his) I bought all those years earlier was also on the shelf at Bodhi Tree.

I decided then and there that my shop would be called breathe books (lowercase B's) and it would be in Baltimore City. I was so excited and totally believed I could do this, as I was learning, through meditation and yoga, that I create my own narrative, my own story, and that truly anything was possible. I called my boyfriend at the time, unable to contain my enthusiasm, and poured out the whole idea. He liked it! Then I walked down Melrose Avenue to a tea shop in West Hollywood and began to write my business plan. Two years later, I opened breathe books. It was successful from day one—everything I had put together fell into place and the Universe provided. I built it, and they came in droves. I ran the store for over a decade—one of the most important decades of my life. I began to more deeply explore Ayurveda *and* I met my husband in that little shop!

In 2004 I saw Deepak Chopra in person for the first time at an Institute of Noetic Sciences (IONS) event in Virginia. By that time, I had read nearly all his books, and felt deeply connected to the teachings within them, which I learned were based on ancient Vedic wisdom from India. In 2007 I attended my first class at the Chopra Center, then located in Carlsbad, California, and my journey into becoming a full-time Ayurvedic counselor, cooking teacher, speaker, and author began.

My Ayurvedic studies coincided with running the bookstore. Customers began to notice that I was different. I had lost weight (and kept it off!), and I was happier and less stressed out. The word "glowing" came up a lot. Ayurveda had transformed me. Eventually, Ayurveda took precedent, and I decided to close my shop and focus my attention fully on working with people to help them establish their Ayurvedic lifestyles.

At its core, Ayurveda and the Vedas are a guide to living in harmony with the seasons and leaning into the natural flow of life. By living in flow with the natural world, we create an alignment that allows us to flourish. In our day-to-day lives, we are often ego-driven, pushing back against what the Universe has presented to us and constantly swimming upstream as we strive to achieve, to make more money, to know important people, and to have more possessions. All this struggle leads us nowhere if we don't feel well, if we are sad, or if we are lonely. Ayurveda teaches the art of flowing downstream, allowing for a natural pace in all stages of our lives.

That's not to say that this flowing is effortless: it takes time, energy, and a willingness to let go and to trust the support of nature's course. Being in balance with the elements in nature means that we must also be in balance with our inner nature. The science and philosophy of Ayurveda gives us a framework to understand nature's cycles, how it moves within us, and how to live in accordance with both of those elements over the course of a day, a season, or entire phases of our lives. And whether through food, meditation, yoga, chanting, aromatherapy, body massage, sleep rituals, breath work, or chakra work, the tried-and-true techniques in this book will help you surely and gently bring yourself back to the best *you* you can be.

Of the many things I have learned over the years, living fully in harmony with the elements is a constant source to my well-being. And it's always there! The hints from Mother Nature are just outside the window, asking you to pay attention, to listen to her, and to make wise decisions accordingly. When we go against our natural urges we create toxic residue in our mind and body, which accumulates and becomes what we call *ama* in Sanskrit. The waste finds its way deep into our tissues and takes hold there, eventually causing disharmony and disease. Ama also affects our thoughts and emotions. When we flow with the cycles of nature—the seasons as well as circadian rhythms, lunar rhythms, and all the other rhythms of life—and work with nature rather than against her, an essence flows through our body called *ojas* (life-enchancing essence). When ojas is flowing freely, we make better choices, have a clearer mind, rarely get sick, and feel attuned and aligned with all beings. I am certain you will find, as I have, that Ayurveda offers a logical and easy-to-follow path to a life full of potential, with tools and techniques available to help you manage whatever arises. Once you know what to look for, Ayurveda has an answer. Let's live in harmony with the seasons and flow down the river of perfect health.

The idea for this book was born out of explorations of themes related to Ayurveda, simmered down to the seasonal nature of the practice. I found there was so much to share! In addition to food, Ayurveda and her sister sciences of meditation and yoga are vast in their ancient wisdom about what can serve us, even today in the modern world. This book is a template for how to adjust your daily life to coincide with nature, creating a deeper sense of awareness of our place in the natural world, and fostering ultimate well-being for your mind and body.

HOW TO USE THIS BOOK

India, where Ayurveda originated, has a different climate than most of us experience in the Northern Hemisphere, where I live. In this book, I have adapted the principles of Ayurveda to a more Western climate, updating the food choices and accounting for our different lifestyles. The basic techniques are all here, with some modern modifications grounded in the theories and concepts I have learned over the years from studying in the US and India, from watching my clients thrive, and from my own experiences as I flow through the stages of life.

Much of Ayurveda focuses on the three doshas, or mind-body types: Vata, Kapha, and Pitta. After you complete the dosha quiz (body and mind) in chapter 2, you will be able to clearly identify which of the three doshas—Vata, Kapha, and Pitta—you are and what imbalances you are currently dealing with. As you become familiar with your own dosha, you will learn how to create a personal seasonal routine by incorporating lifestyle rituals and food recommendations that will align with your unique needs for every day of the year. Whenever you feel lost or out of balance, you can turn to the season and the section you need, based on your individual situation, to discover remedies and recipes, shopping lists, breath work, meditations, mantras, and more, to nudge you back to a state of equilibrium—where you feel clear, focused, satisfied, healthy, and happy.

As you make these changes, be at ease with yourself and start slowly. One of my favorite phrases is "No efforting." Let the changes you make feel natural. Give yourself time. The imbalances that have accumulated in you have had a lifetime to manifest, spread, and become firmly rooted, so it will take some time to shake them lose, shift the balance, remove the obstacles, and begin to feel truly well.

Make incremental adjustments to your routine and watch the benefits unfold. Maybe for you it's best to begin by making an essential oil blend, or by starting to meditate. Or maybe you are ready to clean out the fridge, take the seasonal grocery list to the store, and stock up on the grains, fruits, and veggies of the season, then dig in to some new recipes. Whatever your starting point is, it's the right starting point for you.

You don't have to worry about doing everything "right" or doing it all 100 percent. Just set your intention and let it flow, without self-judgment or criticism. Be kind to yourself and delight in the little changes. These small changes will accumulate, and soon you will be living Ayurveda and feeling terrific.

I urge you to stick with it. Slowly and surely you will see that your sleep becomes deeper, your stress level will be lower, and you will be able to focus more easily even when challenged. Perhaps even illnesses, like diabetes, will reverse, your blood pressure will become normal, and your weight will stabilize. IBS and IBD symptoms may subside. You may even be able to lighten the load of pharmaceuticals you take. I have seen all these things happen for my clients over the years. Turnarounds are not only possible, they are probable. Food is medicine. Breath is medicine. Movement is medicine. You have the power to take control or your life, one action—and one season—at a time.

In the chapters that follow, you will learn how to recognize the attributes of each season, and how they manifest in you. You will learn why we crave more food in winter and less in summer. Why we get bogged down with seasonal allergies, colds, and coughs in spring. And you will learn why like attracts like and how to use the science of opposites to mitigate seasonal ailments with food, drink, movement, the breath, and more.

At the end of the book, you will find the resources to support you on your journey of a lifetime. These seasonal rituals will help you determine when you are hungry and when you are not, what you are craving and why, and how best to take care of your own personal needs throughout the year. You will learn the importance of paying attention to those needs and desires and how to soothe the energy body as well as the physical body. The key is to move slowly and make incremental changes that will last forever.

Baby steps can be a challenge for some people. If you are primarily Pitta dosha, you will want to dive in 100 percent and expect to see changes in weeks if not days. If you don't see a significant metamorphosis, you might be tempted to drop it and say, "Ayurveda isn't for me anyway." Vata may think it's too hard to stick to a routine, and become distracted by the next new thing to come along. Kapha may think, *Well, I know it's good for me, maybe I'll start tomorrow*—but that "tomorrow" never comes.

Each dosha will approach this transformation differently, and I will be there for you—through this book and on my website and in my newsletter—to hold your hand and cheer you on. Simple, small steps will lead to profound changes. Let's begin.

CHAPTER 1

The Roots and Rhythms
of Ayurveda

A yurveda is the oldest medical system in existence. Everything you need to know about how to live life to the fullest is covered in the texts of Ayurveda: the *Charaka Samhita*, the *Sushruta Samhita*, and the *Ashtanga Hridayam*. From surgery to psychiatry, pediatrics to geriatrics, dermatology to ophthalmology— it was all there more than five thousand years ago! The *rishis* (literally "seers")—the great physicians and practitioners who created the field of Ayurveda—promoted a system of living with the elements in nature as well as the elements inside of us. It is a system of balance and harmony with your surroundings and the seasons, based on your unique constitution.

As such, Ayurveda is structured to take your entire being into account. You are much more than your physical and energetic body. You have thoughts, feelings, beliefs, and emotions, which are just manifested outcomes of your experiences. But they feel real and sometimes overwhelming. Ayurveda offers a skilled way of understanding physical and emotional outcomes and managing our reactions to our environment and experiences as they arise. Some of these sensations can be uncomfortable, causing unease in our minds and disease in our bodies. When this occurs, it is nature's way of telling us that something is off-balance and requires attention.

At the core of Ayurveda is a deep recognition of the rhythms of nature. There are times of day for specific rituals, cycles of life for certain actions, and disease-preventing protocols to increase wellness and longevity. Health, well-being, and our lives happen in cycles—and the cycle that most guides and informs our lives is the changing of seasons. The temperature, the weather, the availability of seasonal foods, and our moods and energy levels all fluctuate over the course of the year, influenced by the qualities inherent to the time of year. For this reason, Ayurveda offers many rules, rituals, and remedies to help you stay in rhythm with the season.

Living in harmony with the seasons seems natural, doesn't it? Without even thinking, we change our clothes when the temperature changes, and turn to different food and drinks depending on the time of year, craving hot chocolate in winter but lemonade in summer, for example. Other ancient systems of medicine, too, regard the seasons as one of the fundamental factors in etiology and pathology, and a powerful instrument in the prevention of diseases.[2] When we look to the elements of nature for guidance and support, her rhythms can nourish and sustain us, offering remedies to rejuvenate us and restore us to our most essential, balanced selves.

As it turns out, though, we don't always make the right choices as spring turns to summer and summer to fall and fall to winter. Somewhere along the way, we started wearing sweaters to work in summer, thanks to bone-chilling air conditioning, and sporting short sleeves in winter as the heat pumps out to sweltering levels. We choose to eat watermelon or drink coconut water in winter because the grocery store has it, and sweet potatoes and salsa in summer for the same reason. We don't adjust our sleep patterns as the days lengthen and shorten. Our exercise routines stay the same (active or inactive), and our daily rituals don't take the change in climate or the season into account. When we are out of sync with the natural world, we challenge our natural ability to digest food, emotions, and thoughts. Literally, our gut bacteria, which helps to digest, break down, and assimilate nutrients, does not function properly when we eat out of season and with a lack of diversity. And we wonder why we get colds or the flu in between seasons or allergies get stirred up in spring!

The good news is that it doesn't have to be this way. Much the same way you'd trade out snow boots for flip-flops, adopting seasonally appropriate self-care rituals will keep you feeling your best no matter the time of year. Ayurveda, in her ancient wisdom, offers many ways of balancing the mind and body, based on your individual, unique makeup. With just a few subtle shifts to your routine, you'll find that your sleep will be deep and restorative. Your weight will cease to fluctuate. You will naturally gravitate to the foods that serve you and leave you feeling energized rather than dull or heavy. You will feel enthusiastic and excited about life, not depleted and overwhelmed. By making conscious choices based on your individual needs and the seasons, you're certain to feel more peaceful and content.

Seasons and the Doshic Attributes

While we in the Western world follow four seasons, in Western Ayurveda, there are only three:

VATA: fall, winter
KAPHA: spring
PITTA: summer

Each season is attributed to one of the three doshas, which are a combination of the Five Great Elements (space, air, fire, water, earth). Fall and early winter display the qualities of Vata dosha—dry, changeable, cold. Late winter and spring have the qualities of dampness, heaviness with either rain or snow, as well as new growth—this is known as Kapha. Summer heat is associated with Pitta—fiery, hot, and intense.

The texts of Ayurveda reflect what the great spiritual and scientific thinkers in India, known as rishis, noticed in nature. They saw that the building blocks of the natural world were the Five Great Elements (known as the Pancha Mahabhutas in Sanskrit). These elements are combined and echoed in all living things: plants, animals, ourselves, and in nature. Each person is made up of all the elements, with some predominating more than others. The rishis saw that some people had more air and space (Vata dosha), some more fire and water (Pitta dosha), and others more water and earth (Kapha dosha), and noticed that when a patient was sick, there was too much or too little of an element present, and that created an imbalance in the body. They learned to identify each patient's doshic imbalance, and then recommended treatments, using food, oil massages, and herbal medicines, based on what was needed to create balance.

According to these ancient writings, "All diseases begin at the junctions of the seasons." This is because at these junctures, the seasons overlap. During this overlap, excess dosha that has built up in the previous season needs to be eliminated before the new season begins. For example, in winter we eat heavier food, which works well for us during the cold months. But as spring arrives (Kapha season), with heavy rains and saturated earth, our bodies are still stagnant with the accumulation from winter. For this reason, we must pay extra-special attention to ridding the body of excess Kapha (water and earth). At the juncture of spring and summer, it is imperative to reduce excess Pitta (heat), and between summer and fall, to reduce excess Vata (dryness).[3]

A SCIENCE OF OPPOSITES

As a science of opposites, Ayurveda notes that like attracts like. To create balance and healing, we do the opposite. For example, if the body is too cold, one way to treat it is to eat heavy, warm food. If the mind is too hot, we cool it down with breath work, meditation, or sandalwood oil on the forehead. If the body is heavy, we feed it lighter foods and get it moving more.

When I first began studying Ayurveda in 2007, the science of opposites was one of the most compelling concepts to me. It seems so intuitive! But to really understand the nuance takes some digging. We must acknowledge our own constitution as well as the environment in which we live—and that includes not just our climate, but also the planes and trains we travel on, the houses we live in, the offices where we work, the relationships we create, and the food we eat to sustain us. Every single thing we take in—every morsel of food, every sound, sight, image—every thought and feeling we have, and every situation we find ourselves in has an effect on us, creating either balance or imbalance. That is, it either serves us or it doesn't.

The rishis go on to say that when a body loses its coherence—the ability to make sense of things and stay in balance—it becomes sick. Treatment for every ailment is the reestablishment of order, of understanding. The excess, which is causing the disease, must be removed for health to be fully achieved. Too much or too little of something can cause this imbalance. So to re-create balance, we must find equilibrium. The ancient text explains it like this:

> We treat a disease-ridden man with disease-removing measures, and the depleted man with impletion. We nourish the emaciated and the feeble and we starve the corpulent and the fatty. We treat the man afflicted by heat with cooling measures and heat to him who is afflicted by cold. We replenish body elements that have suffered decrease, and deplenish those that have undergone increase. By treating disorders properly with measures which are antagonistic to their causative factors, we restore the patient to normal.[4]

When we go against the natural order of things, we cause a disruption in the instinctive flow of our health, and plant the seeds of future disharmony or disease. Our goal always (and the aim of this book!) is to guide ourselves gently and naturally back to perfect health—the way we were meant to be.

People of each dosha are affected differently by the elements, their surroundings, and the food they eat. The mind can be brought back into balance with the use of sounds, scents, breathing, meditation, and movement. The body uses food, exercise, and self-massage to establish a vessel for healing and harmony. When both mind and body are in balance, it is easier to make choices that will serve you for the long run.

The more you practice these rituals, the more they will become a natural part of your daily routine. I suggest giving each ritual at least

21 days. That experience will let you begin to see the benefits, reap the rewards, and incorporate them into your life permanently.

ESTABLISHING A SEASONAL ROUTINE

The concept of a seasonal routine is so foundational to Ayurveda that it can be found in the very first chapters of the *Charaka Samhita*. It says, "The strength and complexion of the person knowing the suitable diet and regimen for every season and practicing accordingly, are enhanced." In essence, learning to embrace the wisdom of the ancient teachings and revising them to fit into your current environment can facilitate deep healing—but working these rituals into a seasonal routine will amplify the benefits of any one ritual on its own. We call these personalized regimens *ritucharya*, from the Sanskrit words *ritu*, meaning "seasons," and *charya*, meaning "guidelines."[5] They comprise a wealth of recommendations for maintaining balance of mind, body, and spirit using the many tools available to you such as food, movement, massage, and meditation.

They say that the prevention of "disease"—or, in the language of Ayurveda, "imbalance"—maintains health. If we follow our seasonal self-care routine, we can mitigate the negative effects caused by seasonal change, as well as create harmony by making the best daily choices.[6] Some of the physical benefits of establishing a seasonal routine include avoiding allergies in spring, heat exhaustion in summer, itchy dry skin in late fall, and weight gain in winter, among many other seasonal challenges you may encounter. Emotional upheavals, too, can be handled by an effective ritucharya, especially for people susceptible to seasonal changes such as seasonal affective disorder (SAD) and depression. Just as important, those who suffer from chronic lifestyle diseases like diabetes, obesity, and cancer—which are believed to be a direct result of or exacerbated by an inappropriate relationship with our environment[7]—can expect to see improvement or even reversal of the disease.

A Note on Seasonal Eating

. . . .

"Food is medicine" is a theory employed not only by Ayurvedic *vaidyas* (doctors) but also by Western healthcare advocates, like Hippocrates, who is often quoted as saying, "Let food be thy medicine and medicine be thy food." Somewhere along the way, this brilliant quote has been forgotten by many in the medical profession, who happily substitute pharmaceuticals, or even surgery, for food. But this is changing. More and more people are recognizing that what we put in our mouths not only feeds our bodies, it also heals mind, body, and soul.[8]

Ayurveda takes this a step further, calling our attention to not just what we eat but *when* we eat. Eating nonseasonal food can lead to deep-seated digestive imbalances, which are directly related to emotional and physical imbalances. For this reason we need to continually adjust our eating habits to suit the season we find ourselves in.

There was a time, before the vast network of food supply chains came into being roughly one hundred years ago, that people only ate food that was local and seasonal.[9] We ate what was readily available and shifted our consumption naturally with the season, and our gut adjusted accordingly. Farm-to-table was not just a fancy restaurant concept—it was just the way things were!

The benefits of seasonal eating were detailed in a groundbreaking study published in the journal *Science* in 2017.[10] Researchers discovered that the microbiota of the Hadza people, an ancient forager-hunter-gatherer group in remote north-central Tanzania, reflects the seasonal availability of different types of food.[11] Between seasons, striking differences were observed in their gut microbial communities, and by studying the patterns, researchers noticed a clear cyclical pattern of microbes that directly correlated with the season, with some microbes disappearing entirely, only to reappear when the season turned.

The microbiome affects our entire being—mind and body. It has been estimated that 90 percent of the body's serotonin (a neurotransmitter often called the "happy" chemical because of its role in mood regulation and the feelings of stability and well-being it causes) is made in the digestive tract.[12] If the gut is compromised—either by not eating a variety of healthy foods or eating foods out of season—you may not be producing enough serotonin. This can lead to feeling blue, foggy, out of sorts, unable to sleep well, malaise, inflamed, pained—even clinically depressed.[13]

Nature offers a variety of foods with each season for a reason, and our microbiome has evolved to require seasonal breaks to allow for different nutrients to meet our needs.[14] Eating nonseasonally and relying on the same foods year-round leads to a nondiverse population of bacteria in our gut microbiome, which can make it harder for us to digest certain foods like wheat and lectins, and can also lead to disease.[15]

Still, with all manner of food being available to most of us all the time, it can be difficult to know what is seasonal. Many of us just give up and eat the same thing, every day, season by season. Oatmeal for breakfast, salad for lunch, pizza for dinner. This lack of nutritional diversity can wreck the gut by decreasing the medley of beneficial, seasonal bacteria in the microbiome.

While it takes practice to discern what we're "meant" to be eating in a given season, again, food is our best medicine. The seasonal shopping lists and food guidelines beginning on page 131 are intended to help you on your journey—these will be some of your best, most essential tools to balance your doshas with the seasons.

In addition to guidance and recipes for seasonally appropriate food, Ayurveda employs many self-care rituals you can easily incorporate into your daily routine. Detoxifying body massage, dry brushing, oral care, use of essential oils, chanting mantras, meditation, breath work, chakra toning, yoga, and more will help you maintain balance for your own mind-body constitution.

The ritucharya you will follow is based on the interaction of your dosha type and the current season, with subtle changes for where you are out of balance. To best create your own personal daily routine, take the dosha quiz on page 16 to determine your natural-born Ayurvedic mind-body constitution, as well as identify any current imbalances. Depending on your dosha, different seasons will aggravate or calm your natural constitution, so in addition to universally helpful guidelines for finding balance in each season, you'll find dosha-specific recommendations in each chapter. You will follow the recommendations for the dosha that is currently out of balance (the highest number on your score). For example, if you are in a hot climate and feeling irritable, frustrated, angry, and impatient—best not to eat hot, spicy food! You would follow the guidelines for summer food and daily routine, concentrating on Pitta-reducing choices, which your microbiome will applaud.

This will all make much more sense after you learn more about your own unique dosha in the next chapter, but these techniques should slowly but surely nudge you back in the right direction to your natural-born dosha, where you will flourish.

The chapters that follow will offer you guidance on how to understand yourself in relation to each season and which self-care techniques will help you maintain your well-being throughout the year. With the right ritucharya, you will begin to notice the subtle shifts and learn how you can adjust your routines to seamlessly move from one season to another. When you live in harmony with the elements, subtle yet profound changes will occur, and you will feel better in body, mind, and spirit.

CHAPTER 2

The Doshas:
Your Unique Combination
of the Elements

According to the *Charaka Samhita*, the word "dosha" can be defined as a mistake, dysfunction, error, fault, or disease; an inaccuracy that leads to chaos; or a transgression against the natural order of things. Wow—that sounds dire, doesn't it? Another way to view the doshas is as three energies, or humors, that make up our entire being. These energies can be in a state of equilibrium, or they can be compromised. When the doshas are proportional to our unique constitution, we are in a state of good health. But when there is too much of a particular dosha present, it can tip the balance, and manifest into physical or emotional disease.[1]

The good news is that the actions we take directly impact the excess doshas. With proper diet and lifestyle, we can keep ourselves on track. The result is that we hopefully stay hearty, robust, and able-bodied for a good, long life, but if we do come up against challenges or illness, we will heal more quickly. Once you have the tools in your toolbox, you can pull out what you need when you need it.

We cannot take a measurement of the doshas through a lab test, but we can see them reflected in our physical traits, our spirit, and how we express ourselves on every level. We have given physicality to the doshas by describing Vata as comprising the elements of space and air, Pitta as fire and water, and Kapha as water and earth. In the body we see this as movement (Vata), metabolism (Pitta), and stability (Kapha).

The doshas are believed to circulate in the body and govern physical, mental, and emotional characteristics.[2] As mentioned previously, they also correspond to the seasons:

VATA: fall, winter
KAPHA: spring
PITTA: summer

Each person is a combination of all three doshas, with one or two predominating. You will have all three in different combinations, which may become exacerbated in the corresponding season. Again, this is why we want to adjust our daily rituals accordingly!

You may naturally be a hot, intense, high-energy/active person (Pitta), but lately you have been feeling withdrawn, ambivalent, and lethargic, and have gained weight. This may be caused by depression or not having access to good food, or it may be a slump you fall into every summer when the heat of the day gets you really down. This is Pitta having a Kapha imbalance. So we treat the imbalance by carefully reducing the amount of Kapha in the diet, which should naturally increase the beneficial qualities of Pitta, and hopefully you will begin to feel enlivened and back to your old self. This could be a cyclical condition, so if you know the imbalance is coming, you can meet it head-on and begin your Kapha-balancing routine in spring to mitigate its effects as summer heat rolls around.

If you are feeling balanced—that means no physical ailments, low stress, sleeping well, good elimination, no wild cravings—follow the self-care rituals you can easily fit into your routine, and use the food guidelines based on each season that best corresponds to the current climate where you live. On page 16, you will find a quiz that will help determine your Ayurvedic mind-body constitution, both your current state of being and your innate mind-body constitution. As you probably know, often our mind says one thing and our body another—Ayurveda offers remedies to balance both!

To best understand your doshic imbalance, take this quiz twice. The first time, keep in mind how you have felt or behaved for most of your life. This will be your *prakruti*, or your innate Ayurvedic dosha, the one you were born with. The second time you take the quiz, focus on how you are feeling now. This will be your *vikruti*, or your current state of being.

For example, if you have been a deep sleeper for most of your life but are currently having trouble falling or staying asleep, or have become a light sleeper, for the "sleep patterns/dreams" question, answer "C" on the quiz the first time you take it, then answer "A" the second time around.

You may find you have one dominant doshic expression, or you may be a combination of doshas. Or perhaps you'll find that you rank highest in one dosha on the body quiz but highest in a different dosha on the mind quiz. Not to worry! This happens often, and is perfectly normal.

Even if you are already familiar with your dosha, I encourage you to take this dosha quiz. This particular quiz is designed to focus on your daily activities and the social and relational qualities of your life. It covers more than the basic "large, medium, or small frame" dosha quizzes that you can find on the internet. This quiz takes a deeper look into why you are the way you are. It's the next best thing to visiting an Ayurvedic practitioner! (And if you *do* have a practitioner, take this quiz and present it to them, as it will help them immensely with your treatment protocol.)

DOSHA QUIZ

Body Quiz

BODY SIZE:
A. I am lanky, thin, and bony.
B. I have a medium, muscular body type.
C. I am stocky, thick, and well padded.

WEIGHT:
A. Low body weight. It can be difficult to gain weight.
B. My weight is normal and stable.
C. Heavier than average. It is difficult for me to lose weight.

HAIR:
A. I have dry, frizzy, brittle hair.
B. My hair is thin and fine. I am balding. I turned gray at a young age.
C. I have thick, full, wavy hair. It tends to be a little oily.

SKIN:

A. Thin skin. My veins are visible. I tend toward dry skin and wrinkles.

B. My skin can be reddish in hue and warm to the touch. I am prone to skin problems like eczema, hives, and rashes. I sweat easily.

C. Thick skin. My veins are not visible. My skin feels cold or cool to the touch. It is smooth, slightly oily, with few wrinkles.

EYES:

A. Small, squinty. I tend to look around when talking.

B. Intense and penetrating gaze. I look directly at people when talking.

C. Large, round, and pleasant. I gaze at people warmly.

TONGUE/MOUTH:

A. My tongue is rough and dry, thin and small, with a dark or black coating. I tend to have a dry mouth and dry or cracked lips.

B. My tongue is thin to medium thick, and pointy. It tends to have a reddish or yellowish coating. My mouth feels warm and moist; my lips are thin and reddish.

C. My tongue is large, full, and rounded; it can have a pink or white coating. My lips are smooth, moist, and thick.

JOINTS:

A. My joints are dry and tend to crack; I am not very flexible.

B. I have warm, loose joints; I am flexible.

C. My joints are well lubricated and thickly padded.
Can have fluid buildup.

NAILS:

A. Not able to grow long as they are thin, crack, and split easily, with dry cuticles. My nail beds are whitish with little to no moon.

B. Flexible, soft nails, pinkish nail beds, full moon.

C. My nails are oily and lubricated, strong and thick, and shiny, with a large cuticle. Little to no visible moon.

BOWEL MOVEMENTS:

A. Often constipated. I go 2 or 3 times a week. My stools are hard, dark, dry, and small. No mess, easy to wipe.

B. I usually go 3 to 5 times a day. My stool can be loose and watery, sometimes hot and burning. The color can be yellowish or light brown. Can be hard to clean.

C. I go once or twice a day like clockwork. I have well-formed, large, light brown stools. Sometimes messy and hard to clean.

BODY TEMPERATURE:

A. I feel cold all the time.

B. I run warm or hot in most climates.

C. I am comfortable, if a bit chilly, most of the time, but I don't like cold, damp days.

HUNGER LEVEL:

A. I feel hungry in the morning but forget to eat. I skip meals throughout the day. I feel gassy and bloated after eating.

B. I am ravenous in the morning. If I don't eat when I'm hungry, I feel agitated, angry, stressed out, and frustrated. I digest food quickly.

C. I am not hungry in the morning. I usually eat because the clock says it's time for a meal. My digestion is slow.

SLEEP PATTERNS/DREAMS:

A. I have insomnia; I am a light sleeper and may sleep 2 to 3 hours a stretch. If I wake in the night, I ruminate. It is difficult to get back to sleep. My dreams are about flying, movement, or creativity. I can feel anxious or worried.

B. I can sleep for 4 to 6 hours and feel rested. My dreams are about challenges, chases, competition, or heat and fire. If I wake, I fall back to sleep quickly, or I solve problems or dilemmas.

C. I sleep deeply, sometimes 9 to 10 hours. It can be difficult to wake up. My dreams are vivid and easygoing; romantic, nurturing. I wake to pee and usually fall back to sleep easily.

Mind Quiz

· · · · ·

WHEN STRESSED OUT:

A. I am anxious and worried and forget things. I blame myself when things go wrong. I can talk about it with others but usually cannot pinpoint what is wrong. I can't eat.

B. I am agitated, frustrated, and impatient with others and myself; I tend to blame others. I hold myself and others to high standards.

C. I withdraw to my nest; I usually blame myself or say nothing at all. I tell people I am fine. I eat to soothe myself.

MOOD:

A. I am spontaneous, enthusiastic, and lively. I like change.

B. I am intense and purposeful. I like to convince people. I get easily frustrated with others. I like things to go my way.

C. I am easygoing and like routine. I like to nurture and support, sometimes at the cost of not caring for myself.

SOCIAL:

A. I tend to be easily distracted and run late. It doesn't bother me if others are late. I have a lot of friends.

B. I am precise and always on time, or a little early. I become distressed and angry when others are not on time. I have a few really good friends.

C. I tend to run late because I move slowly. I overthink the situation and that causes me to be late. I don't mind if I have to wait for others. I have many friends, but not all of them are good for me.

HOME:

A. I like a bright, sunny household, with few items. I toss extra things away. I like it spare, clean, colorful, and functional.

B. I like a neat home with fine, top-of-the-line items. I have high-quality art, electronics, furniture, and clothes.

C. I like to nest. "Shabby chic" describes my style. I have a lot of clutter but it doesn't bother me too much. I rarely throw things away, as I feel attached to things long after they are no longer useful.

MONEY:

A. I don't keep track of my spending. If I like something, I buy it, but I don't always have a use for it. I don't have a budget in mind when I spend. I do not save or invest, or I do so sporadically.

B. I keep a tight budget but will always spend top dollar for quality products. I spend money on goods and services. I spend as needed when I want something. I invest money, sometimes on risky propositions.

C. I like to spend money on myself, spas, vacations, good restaurants. I really enjoy spending money on experiences. I save money for a rainy day. I invest for the long term.

WORK ROUTINE:

A. I get easily distracted at work or while doing everyday tasks. I need others to help keep me on track or things don't get finished.

B. I am intense and focused on my tasks. I don't leave the job until it is finished to my satisfaction. I prefer to work alone or direct others under me.

C. I am happy to work on projects with others. I work slowly and steadily, but get the job the done.

CREATIVITY:

A. I am highly creative and always thinking of new things to make or design. I begin many projects and often do not follow through to completion.

B. I like researching new challenges and directing a team to get the job done. I always complete what I begin, or I delegate it to someone else.

C. I love to go to museums, art shows, and concerts, but I don't have the energy to create much myself.

Prakruti (birth dosha) score:

BODY:
A: _____ B: _____ C: _____

MIND:
A: _____ B: _____ C: _____

Vikruti (current state dosha) score:

BODY:
A: _____ B: _____ C: _____

MIND:
A: _____ B: _____ C: _____

MOSTLY A = VATA DOSHA
MOSTLY B = PITTA DOSHA
MOSTLY C = KAPHA DOSHA

SCORING YOUR QUIZ

Total up your A's, B's, and C's for the way you have been most of your life: this is called your prakruti. Your prakruti is determined at birth—it's your innate, natural-born mind-body constitution, which is a combination of actions that occur before, during, and after conception. Depending on the state of mind of your parents, the food they ate, the circumstances surrounding your conception and birth (the location, climate, and season, the food and drink and substances your mother took in during pregnancy)—all come into play to create the person you are. Once you are aware of your prakruti, either through this dosha quiz or by working with an Ayurvedic practitioner, it is important not to let that definition limit you. Rather, use it as a tool to understand your own unique way of expression, personal development, quirks, traits, and your individual presence in the world.

Only by understanding, appreciating, and embracing your true nature can you truly thrive. The goal is not to change your prakruti (you can't, anyway!) but rather to embody the balanced attributes of the dosha. For example, Vatas can learn to manage energy rather than wasting it and becoming depleted, exhausted, and weak. Pittas can harness their heat and, rather than competing and being single-mindedly driven toward success, they can use their warmth to teach, mentor, and be an effective leader. Kaphas can learn ways to let go of things they accumulate (and that hold them back), and instead use their innate gifts of stability, support, and caring to nuture themselves and others.

The second time you take the quiz—for your current state of mind and body—you will discover your vikruti. When we are born, we enter into a world of unknowns, and the body and mind begin to adjust to the new reality outside of the comfort of the womb. This can cause deep changes to your prakruti, resulting in specific concerns, struggles, or disorders that you are currently facing. This is where we will start—with changes in your daily life, based on the season, to diminish any glaring obstacles in your way. Once we have your vikruti under control, you will return to maintaining balance in your prakruti.

These imbalances don't always show up right at birth. They can appear many years later as we go through our different stages of life, and they tend to show up in one of two ways. You may find that you're experiencing an excess of your natural dosha—too much of a good thing can make us out of balance with ourselves. For example, an infant whose prakruti is Vata, who has been born into a calm, stable household, in a humid, warm climate, might be curious, happy, interested, highly attuned to their environment, and keen to engage. Their Vata is stable. But a Vata infant can also be slightly lower weight, longer limbed, highly alert, and active, a finicky eater, and a light sleeper. If that child is born into a chaotic, loud, arid, and cold household devoid of routines—like eating and sleeping on a schedule—they will likely become unstable, displaying the qualities of an out-of-balance Vata child. The result could be a highly creative being that is easily distracted, scared, and fearful, who is often sick and can't sit still or pay attention. Their vikruti is Vata, out of balance. The telltale signs for Vata out of balance are anxiety, fear, and worry.

Alternatively, a Kapha infant is typically easygoing, playful, and a deep sleeper, and is usually a bit more roly-poly than the other doshas. If this happy, sweet-natured child is born into an angry household with yelling and conflict, and does not feel cared for or tended to, this infant could begin to display Pitta imbalances—screaming and crying, becoming red in the face, swatting things away, inconsolable with hunger. This child will have a vikruti of Pitta—angry, frustrated, impatient.[3]

Taking a good look at who you are, based on your reactions, your mood, and your physical traits—these will tell you your vikruti.

If your prakruti and vikruti are different, you will first want to use this book to balance your highest score on the vikruti quiz.

Regardless of the season, you can choose the foods and routines to pacify that imbalance. For example, if you are having migraines and hives and it's December, try using the summer-reducing routine until these Pitta-like symptoms disappear, and then return to the winter routine. In other words, cool down the Pitta, then return to the Vata routine.

If you're experiencing an imbalance of . . .

VATA: follow guidelines for fall/winter (page 37)
KAPHA: follow guidelines for spring (page 69)
PITTA: follow guidelines for summer (page 99)

If your prakruti and vikruti are the same or the numbers are close, follow recommendations for your prakruti. This will help you to maintain mind-body balance.

Remember, while we all have all three doshas, your ultimate goal is *not* to be tri-doshic—which is very rare—but rather to be the best representation of your primary dosha that you can be. If you are truly equally balanced with Vata, Pitta, and Kapha, that can be a beautiful way to navigate the seasons. Often, though, if you are tri-doshic, when it's too cold and dry, our Vata is out of whack. If it is too hot and humid, your Pitta will erupt. If it's damp and cold, your Kapha will accumulate.

But if you generally feel good and healthy, and your dosha quiz does reflect more or less equal amounts of Vata, Pitta, and Kapha, you can use this book by following the seasonal guidelines without regard to a specific doshic imbalance. Of course, if you begin to notice something is out of balance, you will have the knowledge for how to adjust your plan to come back to your natural state of being.

BALANCING YOUR DOSHAS

To review, the Pancha Mahabhutas, or "Five Great Elements," are space, air, fire, water, and earth. Each dosha is a combination of the elements:

VATA = SPACE AND AIR
PITTA = FIRE AND WATER
KAPHA = WATER AND EARTH

The doshas cycle with the seasons, from accumulation to aggravation to calmative—as a season progresses, we accumulate too much stuff, it disagrees with us, and then we have to get rid of it to feel better once again! But we need each dosha to be working well in order for our body to function properly.

We need Vata for movement and circulation, Pitta for digestion and metabolism, and Kapha to keep us supported and stable. We feel our best when we balance our inner elements with the elements in nature. It is for this reason that Ayurveda works so closely with the seasons. That alignment is the sweet spot where you are in complete harmony with your surroundings.

It is important to know, however, that your dosha does not define who you are. I often tell my clients to use the knowledge of the doshas as a guidepost, then just forget about it and live seasonally, coming back to the guidepost as needed. We all love to define ourselves one way or another—but Ayurveda is not a Myers-Briggs test or an Enneagram. It is a road map to a deeper understanding of why you are the way you are, and to learn to nurture, feed, and care for yourself based on those needs, for prevention and longevity. Basically, it's about growing old well. Know thy dosha, know thyself, and move on!

Vata Characteristics
• • • • • • • • • • •

ELEMENTS: Space and Air

TRAITS: Vata dosha is light and thin with dry skin and hair, and cold hands and feet. Vata is hyperactive and restless, a light sleeper with a low sex drive. Vata loves trying new things, is easily distracted, resists routine, forgets to eat, spends money without consideration, and is very creative. Vata likes cold, raw, bitter, sour, and dry foods.

QUALITIES:

- Changeable
- Cold
- Light
- Dry
- Fast

- Irregular
- Rough
- Spontaneous
- Talkative
- Mobile

COMMON AILMENTS: When stressed out, Vata tends to blame themselves, become confused, forget to eat, and cannot sleep. They ruminate, causing high anxiety and needless worry. Vata ailments include constipation; dry skin; arthritis; dry eyes; brittle nails; dandruff; manic depression; severe joint problems; tremors; IBS and IBD; weak constitution.

WHEN BALANCED:

- Good communicator
- Speaks their mind
- Adaptable
- Visionary
- Innovative
- Original
- Productive
- Prolific
- Original
- Energetic

WHEN OUT OF BALANCE:

- Anxious
- Worried
- Fearful
- Mentally irritated
- Insomniac
- Difficult digestion
- Constipated
- Inconsistent
- Often runs late
- Forgets to eat

Pitta Characteristics

• • • • • • • • • •

ELEMENTS: Fire and Water

TRAITS: Pitta dosha is typically medium to strong build, with hair that turns gray and thins early. They are warm-blooded, sweat easily, and have a very strong sex drive. Pitta doesn't need much sleep (and loves to tell everyone!). They have strong digestive fires and gravitate toward spicy foods. Pitta is very smart, learns quickly, and is direct, precise, and courageous. They are good communicators and speakers, love routine, and tend to spend money on high-end, fancy objects.

QUALITIES:

- Hot
- Acidic
- Fiery
- Intense
- Sharp
- Penetrating
- Light
- Pungent

COMMON AILMENTS: When stressed out, Pitta blames others, lashes out, and fires back. They also can hold themselves accountable if they feel they were not living up to their own high standards. Pitta ailments include rosacea; fever; migraines; excessive sweating; herpes/shingles; anorexia; prostate issues; heartburn; GERD; acid reflux; burning eyes; hives.

WHEN BALANCED:

- Friendly
- Warm
- Quick decision-maker
- Healthy digestion
- Persuasive
- Personable

WHEN OUT OF BALANCE:

- Mean
- Angry
- Petty
- Blames others
- Perfectionistic
- Judgmental
- Hypercritical
- Harsh
- Alienating
- Aggressive
- Intimidating
- Cruel

Kapha Characteristics
· · · · · · · · · · ·

ELEMENTS: Water and Earth

TRAITS: Kapha tends to be heavier than the other doshas, with thick skin and well-lubricated, padded joints. They can have a sweet, melodious voice; large eyes; thick hair and skin; large, white teeth; and full lips. Kapha is a deep sleeper, and likes to sleep long hours—sometimes ten or more. They have a steady sex drive and are very sensuous people. Kapha gains weight easily and has difficulty losing it. They have great stamina and rarely get sick. Kapha loves sweet, sour, salty, creamy, and rich foods.

QUALITIES:

- Heavy
- Slow
- Sluggish
- Slimy
- Smooth
- Stable
- Cold
- Solid
- Watery

COMMON AILMENTS: When stressed out, Kapha withdraws and would rather not deal with things. They will eat, nest, and sleep. Ailments affecting Kapha include obesity; high cholesterol; wet cough; excess phlegm; bronchitis; allergies; sinus infection; low appetite; lethargy.

WHEN BALANCED:

- Caring
- Warm
- Content
- Easygoing
- Loves to please
- Patient
- Lovable
- Enjoys a routine
- Saves money
- Very thoughtful
- Stable

WHEN OUT OF BALANCE:

- Congested
- Heavy
- Dull
- Inert
- Greedy
- Needy
- Overly protective
- Collector/hoarder
- Hermit
- Stuck

We move through the doshas in the stages of our lives as well as through the seasons on the calendar. As you learn more about your dosha, you will see why you feel better at certain times of year and out of balance at others. One season is your friend, another your enemy. For example, Pitta dosha feels at home in the summer, which fuels their Pitta fire. But they will notice that too much heat can cause serious problems in the mind and body: migraines, heat rash, hives, and indigestion in the physical body, and anger, irritability, and frustration in the mind. This is why many Pittas prefer the winter. The cold air helps to keep the excess fire in check. You may see these folks in T-shirts and shorts on cold, windy winter days. And they are loving it!

Vata dosha, on the other hand, can really suffer in winter—their hands and feet never seem to get warm enough, and no matter how many layers they have on, they can still feel chilled to the bone. But they love big sweaters and blankets and soft socks, which ground and soothe the Vata soul—lending a sense of security and safeness. Summer is truly their favorite time of year, when they finally begin to thaw out! Taking off the layers from winter and spring, they find a new sense of freedom and movement.

Kapha loves winter, when eating more is appropriate and sleeping in is not frowned upon. But when springtime comes around, Kapha begins to accumulate fluid and mucus, and everything stagnates. If they allow themselves to become too laid-back and dismissive of self-care in winter, they will find themselves severely compromised as spring rolls around. To kaphic people, Kapha season is the enemy. Sinus congestion, allergies, bronchitis, and sinusitis can occur. The air can still be cold, but the earth begins to produce new growth from increased rain, creating muddy ground and setting the stage for discomfort in the Kapha mind and body. The drying winds but still-warm temperatures of early fall—Vata season—should be Kapha's best friend. Excess fluids begin to dry up, the warm air melts away fat that may have accumulated in winter and spring, and the overall quality of letting go of excess earth (mud and water) has a soothing, reducing quality on Kapha. They feel light and invigorated.

When I take a look back at my life, I see the doshic stages clearly. As a young child in the mid-1960s and early 1970s I see such a Vata-Kapha person—meaning I was carefree and easily distracted, and felt loved and secure. I would run around our neighborhood like a cheerful flower child. Not a care in the world. Curly hair flying. Rolling in the grass. Unselfconscious. Putting on plays with my two older sisters, singing show tunes and popular music. Drawing colorful and messy pictures—staying in the lines was not my forte! I made friends easily— my mother used to say I could make a friend even if I was in a box. I remember being a very active, happy-go-lucky child. The Vata in me was breezy and spontaneous. The Kapha felt held, secure, loved, and supported. I had a stable playground to explore all the possibilities around me.

As I hit puberty, I began to put on weight and became self-conscious, and maybe a little angry and rebellious (my mom would probably say a lot rebellious!). That was Kapha and Pitta—the elements of excess water and earth—creating a heavier, curvier frame, and the fire of puberty igniting my emotions and reactions. As the hormones began to rage, I definitely entered a more turbulent phase—never taking "no" for an answer. Determined to get my own way. Stubborn, fearless, and headstrong. Maybe even a bit reckless. Pitta all the way.

Eventually, the Pitta phase calmed down and my Vata-Kapha nature took over. I was not one to stay in one place for a long period of time (Vata moves like the wind). I traveled around the world (Vata) and easily made friends and landed smoothly (Kapha loves to nest). I had the most interesting jobs but never really strived for high positions or money (low Pitta—not type A in the least). I was often distracted by shiny new objects (Vata), but was able to make steady work out of those diversions (Kapha—slow and steady wins the race).

I could be spontaneous in thought and diligent in practice—so Vata-Kapha!

Now, as I am settling into the other side of menopause, after experiencing physical and emotional hot flashes—a return to Pitta Pitta Pitta!—I find the heat subsiding, and a full-blown Vata taking over; this is the natural progression of the doshas as we age. The urge to create, try new things, and move from one project to another has felt freeing and exciting. The Vata years can be incredibly uplifting and adventurous as the constraints of expectations (if indeed you ever felt them) are gone, and you can make your days into anything you want.

As you can see, the doshas are not just manifested in your body, but also in your mind, and they define your stage of life. Additionally, the doshas are in the time of day, as well as in each season. Doshas are also present in our bodily tissues in the form of illness and disease, and in different organs at various stages of accumulation. While we cannot measure the doshas through scientific means, we can begin to notice increased manifestations as we educate ourselves on how, why, and where they present themselves.

It is amazing to see the doshas in ourselves and how they can rule our lives. How have the doshas played a role in the unfolding of your life? Look back on your decisions and see if you can pinpoint which dosha helped to steer you and how it manifested. As you begin to add some of the self-care rituals into your routine, you will watch your life expand with ease, with a sense of joy and happiness. Just as the seasons of the year form a system to help us remember how to care and feed ourselves, the seasons of our lives offer challenges, reminders, and rewards at every stage. By living in harmony with your natural life cycle as well as the cycles of the year, you will be naturally fulfilled, living a life of true balance, acceptance, and ease of being.

CHAPTER 3

Vata Season (Fall/Winter)

VATA
. . .

Air and Space. Late fall through early winter. Digestive fire is burning bright. Focus on staying warm and lubricated. Eat hearty, warm, cooked foods.

. . .

QUALITIES:
changeable, dry, cold, light (late fall, early winter);
heavy (late winter)

ELEMENTS:
space, air, earth

DOSHAS MOST AFFECTED:
Vata in the late fall and early winter, Kapha late winter

TASTES TO FAVOR:
sweet, sour, salty

TASTES TO AVOID:
bitter, pungent, astringent

COMMON AILMENTS:
depression; lethargy; colds and flu;
cold hands and feet; joint pain; dry skin

DAILY BODY MASSAGE:
warm, calming, grounding sesame seed oil,
almond oil, or mustard seed oil

. . .

In late fall and early winter, we can feel the sun begin to recede from the earth, taking with it the heat of summer. Soon we begin to see chilly winds, whipping leaves off the trees just as they turn to beautiful shades of autumn colors. A cold and dry climate takes form, changing day to day from warm, to hot, to cold, before the heavy snows or rains of late winter take place. These are all the attributes of Vata—cold, dry, changeable, rough, quick, and irregular. When we see these changes in nature, we can begin to turn to remedies, foods, and daily routines to help us stay warm and grounded.

We want to bring the opposite qualities into our daily rituals to counterbalance those attributes. That means dressing in layers, eating hot, cooked foods, drinking warm liquids, and keeping the body well oiled—inside and out.

The shortening days from fall through midwinter also offer more time to rest, to settle in and slow down. As the sun sets we can aim for an earlier dinner and earlier bedtime. The abundant growth from summer goes fallow, dries up, and withers away. We see a reduction in summertime activities, less time outdoors, and a shift in the foods we crave. In winter, we are naturally hungrier, longing to dig into hearty, satisfying, warming foods, as our *agni* (digestive fires) burns brighter, causing us to feel hungrier. For some, putting on a few pounds of winter weight can to keep us warm and grounded.

Winter offers a unique opportunity to be still, go within, reflect, and recalibrate. The cold, short days are ideal for ending the evening early, waking just before sunrise, and taking time for contemplation. By slowing down, perhaps we can see more clearly what is important and what is best left behind. Try not to let yourself become dull and inert during this season. Use the chill in the air to enliven you, increase activity, and bring new practices into your life.

Through slow, deep breath work, you feel safe and secure. Your meditation practice will be still and quiet as the mornings are dark, allowing you to be still, present, and focused. Our daily routine rituals will keep the body oiled, smooth, and lubricated, which in turn helps the mind to stay settled. And the food you choose will contain a variety of tastes, colors, and nutrients to keep you healthy and well-fed through the season.

By following the guidelines detailed here, each dosha can stay more or less balanced during the season. Remember to be good to yourself, begin to make changes slowly, and take baby steps. Slow and steady is the best way to incorporate these changes into your *dinacharya*, or daily routine. You can begin by just choosing one or two things each day, or even each week. By the end of the season you will have made plenty of changes, and you will begin to see how beneficial these suggestions can be.

DINACHARYA FOR VATA SEASON

Eat ....

There are no two ways around it: winter is a season focused on food. We can see this in all of nature: In late fall I watch squirrels outside my office window busily scurrying around, looking for places to bury their nutritious acorn nuggets, as they know they will need all those juicy calories in the coming months. My dogs also begin to eat more—even my notoriously picky border collie mix, Ella (full name Ellananda Shakti Weis-Bohlen), is eager for breakfast to arrive.

We crave warm, hearty food because agni—our digestive fire—is the highest in this season. Ayurveda says our bodies were designed this way so that we have fuel for the fire to keep us warm. We need to keep the fire burning bright in our bellies to give us the energy needed to stay nourished during the cold months. Agni is like a fireplace—a few strategically placed logs creates a beautiful, bright fire. Then there is the temptation to add another log, then another, and before you know it, the fire is smothered. Simply put: Don't eat too much or you will put out the fire! Agni helps to burn *ama*—literally "undigested food." And to increase *ojas*—a vital essence within us that boosts our immune system and supports vitality, longevity, and mental and physical health. Ojas is the lightness we feel when healthy, dosha-appropriate food, as well as good thoughts, emotions, images, and sensations, are absorbed deeply into our tissues, pushing toxins out. This is how nutrients are assimilated and waste is eliminated.

In the colder months, agni is burning bright so the appetite is high. If we eat until we are just 80 percent full, the fires keep burning, our food is properly digested, and we feel energetic and satisfied. The temptation is there, however, to add more fuel to the flame—in the form of food and drink. So, you have a few more bites, a bit of dessert, a latte, or an after-dinner drink. And boom—the flame is tamped out and you feel dull, inert, tired—couch potato. Try to catch yourself before you overeat, especially in this season when the urge to indulge is great. In Ayurveda we say when you burp, you are done. So pay attention! You may have to push that food away before your mind says it's full, but your body has let you know it's over.

The trick of this season will be to choose food that is satisfying on every level and that will reduce cravings. Ayurveda says to have six tastes in every meal—sweet, sour, salty, pungent, bitter, and astringent. In the colder months, sweet, sour, and salty (the most densely nutritive foods) help to balance us during Vata season—but don't forget the other tastes! A winter spice blend, or *churna* (page 42 or 142), is easy to add to any food and is a simple way to incorporate the other flavors into your diet.

VATA SEASON SPICE MIX

1 tablespoon coriander seeds

1 tablespoon cumin seeds

2 tablespoons fennel seeds

2 tablespoons ground ginger

1 tablespoon ground turmeric

1 tablespoon dried basil

1 teaspoon sea salt

1/2 teaspoon hing (asafœtida)

Combine all the spices in a spice grinder or clean coffee grinder and grind. Spoon the ground spice mix into a clean glass jar or stainless-steel container with a lid. Make sure there is a tight seal on the container. The spices contain essential oils that we want to keep stable. Best used within 1 year to ensure the freshness of the healing properties in the spices. Store in a cool, dark place. You can fill a small jar to carry with you when you go out.

In the winter, it is essential for Vata and Pitta to eat three meals a day, but to avoid snacking, in all seasons, if possible. Your body digs deep into the stored pockets of energy between meals to keep you going. This is how we burn fat and reduce toxins. Vata dosha, in particular, may need more food—they tend to space out if they don't stick to a strict eating schedule—so be aware of your hunger level and feed yourself before you become famished. If you must snack, nuts, seeds, and sweet fruits or fresh cheese or other high-protein foods are a good choice for Vata dosha in the winter.

Kapha dosha, on the other hand, can do very well on two meals a day, avoiding snacks altogether. All doshas should have their largest meal between ten a.m. and two p.m., as this is Pitta time of day, when the sun is the highest, offering us a natural boost in digestion.

Your activity levels are likely to be lower in the winter, so we need to make sure the body is sufficiently fueled at meal times and given a metabolic rest between, which some people call intermittent fasting. In all seasons, it is an excellent post-meal ritual to take a 10-minute walk to help the agni stay stoked. This keeps the blood circulating to enhance digestion. If you feel too tired or lethargic, that means you probably overate. You can do better next time. One should feel energized and alert after a good meal, not stuffed and dull.

Note: Intermittent fasting is not for everyone. If you have diabetes or are on medications for diabetes, have a history of eating disorders (binge eating, anorexia, or bulimia), or are pregnant or breastfeeding, you should consult your primary care practitioner before starting an intermittent fasting diet.

All doshas should also sip warm water with your meals. We often forget to stay hydrated when it's cold outside, but overheated office buildings, or going from a heated car to a heated store or restaurant can really dry you out. Never drink iced cold drinks, especially with food; they will put out your agni. Instead, keep warm water close at hand, ideally with a squeeze of lemon for Kapha and Vata, or lime for Pitta and drink a few ounces before your meal to get the digestive juices moving. When you are out during the day, carry a travel mug filled with hot water and a few slices of fresh ginger. Sip this throughout the day instead of coffee, sugary beverages, or cold drinks. (My favorite travel mugs are made of stainless steel, which will keep your beverages hot for hours!) It will not only help to keep you warm, but warm/hot water is better absorbed by your tissues and will keep you hydrated all day long in those hot, dry offices, cars or train, stores—even at home.

WINTER TEA BLEND

Drinking hot tea in cold weather will gently warm you from the inside out. We concentrate on sweet tastes—like cinnamon and cardamom, as well as ginger and licorice. You can make you own blend or buy one ready-made. Adding a dollop of milk or a natural nut- or coconut-based nondairy creamer can really make your drink special.

Another is the famous Ayurvedic tea called CCF tea. "CCF" stands for cumin, coriander, and fennel seeds. Steep 1/2 teaspoon of each in a pot of 3 to 4 cups hot water. Pour through a strainer and enjoy! I use the same seeds two or three times.

Intelligent use of food is crucial, especially at the cusp of the season. If you are not able to do anything else, at least simplify your diet as we move into winter. That means avoiding processed, fried, overly sweet, and super-rich foods. Choose simple, easy-to-digest foods with few ingredients. Avoid raw, cold foods. Foods that are cold, raw, processed, and heavy in sugar and salt are harder to digest, robbing your body of the energy it needs to keep you warm and to stave off the flu, colds, sore throat, and other winter ailments. Leave the salads for the warmer months. However, if you must eat cold food, at least sip warm water or herbal tea with it. Sauté your greens, or top your salad with some hot rice, millet, or quinoa and beans or steamed vegetables.

During the workday, make adjustments so that you can eat your food hot. Warm food is so much more satisfying than a cup of yogurt or a sandwich. In order to avoid the potentially detrimental aspects of using the microwave (in Ayurveda, we say that intense heat diminishes the prana—the life-force—of the food), you can take soup or stew to work in a camping thermos. Just heat your food up on the stove in the morning, put it in your thermos, and leave it on your desk until lunchtime. Your food will be nourishing, yummy, and warm.

The Eating Out Challenge

I stopped eating meat when I was sxiteen years old. I really didn't know much about nutrition, but I had a job at the juice bar of a health food store called Nature's Cupboard, so I learned how to make many recipes: avocado cheese melts, peanut butter with honey and bananas, cauliflower casseroles, powerhouse sandwiches with Havarti cheese and vegan mayo. Most of this food was fatty and yummy. It's no wonder my weight was teetering in the 180-pound zone. If someone asked me about being vegetarian back then, I would have said it's all pizza, pasta, and peanut butter!

One of the frequent customers at my juice bar was Oprah Winfrey, who was then a reporter at our local TV station, WJZ. Oprah would come in, sit at the juice bar, and gab with us after jogging around the complex—we loved her. She was trying to lose weight even back then (1980). We all thought snacking on carob-covered almonds and drinking carrot juice would help us! We didn't know anything about Ayurveda, combining foods, the six tastes, or agni and ojas. If it was in a health food store, it must be good for you, right? Needless to say, none of us lost weight or got much healthier in those days.

Many, many years later, with my Ayurvedic education in my back pocket, I am much wiser when I eat out of the house (and I think Oprah is, too!). Most chefs are not trained in nutrition or focused on making your meal extra healthy—after all, their specialty is flavor, usually meaning more salt—so it is often up to us to put together a healthy meal.

During the winter months, I cook most of our meals at home and go out less often. I recommend that my clients do the same. Though, of course, you can do this in any season, something about it seems easier when we're already less inclined to venture outside into the cold. Instead of meeting friends for coffee or dinner, have them over for tea or make a pot of soup to share. Not only is it healthier, you may find that you enjoy the communion of sharing a meal in your own home.

If you must eat out, I recommend that you graze several side dishes instead of one entrée. The sides are often much healthier—greens, potatoes, grains, and beans. Soup and some sides makes for a perfectly satisfying meal. You can even ask the server to put the sides together on one plate to make it look like an entrée and have it served alongside all the other entrées, if you are eating with others. It really makes a difference. And don't be shy about asking for what you want and bringing your own condiments. Some restaurants use very cheap, unhealthy (I would say even deadly) vegetable oil. Bring your own organic oil—ghee, extra-virgin olive, safflower, sunflower—and ask the server to request that the chef use this for your meal, if it contains oil. You can say you have an allergy (an allergy to bad oil!). I also want to encourage you to bring your own spice churna (see recipes in each season) along with you. These mixes will not only make your food tastier, they will also enhance your digestion. You can fill just a small jar or shaker and take it with you when you eat out.

A Note on Holiday Eating
. . . .

From September to January there seems to be one holiday after another, and they all seem to be focused on food.
With Rosh Hashanah, the Jewish New Year, there are apples
dipped in honey. Halloween candy comes around the corner,
then Thanksgiving pumpkin pie, sweet potatoes with toasted
marshmallows, and pecan pie. Hanukkah brings latkes and
oil-laden food, and Christmas, well, do not even get me started
on holiday cookies! At the end of the year, Kwanzaa culmi-
nates with the Karamu feast—collards, catfish, and a variety of
hearty dishes. The abundance of this season is truly delicious,
but why throw away an entire year of making good choices
just for a sugar high to get us through the winter? Health is
not a seasonal state of being. It should be considered a way of
life, every day of the year.

Food is such a huge part of our seasonal traditions and
rituals. Following Ayurvedic guidelines for the season doesn't
mean that you can't enjoy meals with family and friends. We
can make choices based on what we feel we need at the time
(which might not always be the best choice), but if we live a
relatively healthy lifestyle, by reducing processed foods, meat,
sugar, and unhealthy fats, we can indulge from time to time.
I've even included a few favorite holiday recipes on pages
143–145. Additionally, moving the body by walking, doing
yoga, or more vigorous exercise and getting plenty of good
sleep can help us more easily recover from a bout of the mun-
chies or even a full-on binge.

Sleep...
Oh, the urge to just dive into a pile of blankets and bury our heads is
great in wintertime. I often find my dogs "making" their bed by push-

ing layers of the blankets on top of each other and settling down in the middle, digging out a little space for their noses to stay warm. I can certainly relate—it's sometimes a fight for the comforter!

It is natural to feel tired when the sun goes down; after all, our circadian rhythm is innate. We want to pay keen attention to what the body is telling us. When you feel tired, go to sleep—don't force yourself to stay awake! Listen to your body. It's dark. Time to wind down and perform a few bedtime rituals to help us sleep well and wake refreshed—even if we are getting up to a dark sky.

Winter allows us the pleasure of going to bed early—take advantage of this as your body needs more time to process the heavier food we take in during this season. Aiming for nine or nine thirty p.m. is good. Taking a warm bath with calming essential oils like vanilla, sandalwood, or lavender is an excellent remedy to help promote a deep sleep. Applying bhringraj oil (an herbal remedy that is not only great for sleep, it's also great for your hair!) to feet and scalp just before bed helps to deeply relax the nervous system, and jotting a few notes in a journal can help to get out any nagging thoughts that are on your mind.

You should also avoid engaging in detailed work like spreadsheets or bank balances—this will greatly disturb the mind. Instead, watch a light movie or show, read something you enjoy, and generally avoid taking on anything taxing or disturbing.

If we are not following specific Vata-balancing techniques, our sleep may be scattered, ungrounded, and fitful, with periods of wakefulness in the night, usually between two and six a.m., which is Vata time of night. If you do wake up during this time, try some relaxing deep breaths, counting the inhale to 5 and the exhale to 6. This is a great sleep aid called vagus nerve breathing. The vagus nerve travels from the brain down through neck through the torso to the abdomen, where it provides stimulation to internal organs and transmits information about the state of those organs to the central nervous system. Regulating and supporting your vagus nerve is essential to both mental and physical relaxation, and during these long, dark winter months, activating the vagus nerve can be a safeguard against depression, seasonal affective disorder, and anxiety. It engages the parasympathetic nervous system, which should help you fall back to sleep. If this does not work, try a mindfulness meditation practice or listen to a meditation app (but don't get caught up looking at your phone!) for sleep.

A healthy night's sleep begins with a healthy bedroom. Remove TVs, computers, iPads, even your phone, if possible, from your room. The electromagnetic frequencies (EMFs) from these electronics can stimulate your brain, as they are never really switched off. In my home we have our Wi-Fi on a timer. It goes off completely at eleven p.m. and turns back on at seven a.m. Try this for a week or so and see if you notice the difference—I'm thinking you will!

Vastu Shastra for Better Sleep

Ayurveda relies on the system of *vastu shastra* (older than but similar to feng shui) for the proper placement and direction of objects to promote health and healing—physically and emotionally. It is an incredibly complex system, but you may find some benefits from a few pointers:

1. For a deep sleep, the head of your bed should be toward east or south. If this doesn't work, try any direction except north.
2. Keep the room free of clutter, especially under the bed.
3. Do not have a mirror at the foot of the bed.
4. Use soft, cool colors on the walls and ceiling, sheets, and covers.
5. If you have a bathroom attached to the bedroom, keep the door closed and the toilet seat down.

6. Avoid having photos of people who have passed away on display.
7. Do not keep a large pile of books next to the bed.
8. Clear the clutter out from bedside tables and under the bed.
9. If you cannot avoid having a TV or computer in the room, cover them with a beautiful scarf or shawl before bedtime.
10. Do not sleep under a beam.

All these precautions have to do with allowing the prana or chi—energy—to flow freely during the night. The body goes through a restorative phase while you are sleeping, and if any of the above are present in the room it will disturb this process. Do what you can and try to clean up your space.

Also disturbing to sleep is having a heavy meal less than three hours before bed. All doshas do well with a small dinner, avoiding too much spice and fat. Vata and Pitta may require a bit more protein than Kapha—keep it light but still substantial, warm, and satisfying. Try not to eat after dinner.

Keep your bedtime consistent, as well as the timings of your meals. The mind will be more at ease if it knows what to expect. Winter can increase anxiety and worry, which spills over from the day into the night, so keeping a routine helps to calm this reaction. Drinking a cup of hot tea before bed is a great way to wind down. Choose a calming herbal tea like lavender, lemon balm, chamomile, or valerian. You may also find taking the supplement ashwagandha, an adaptogenic herb, to be very useful for inducing sleep. Sip your tea, make some notes in your journal, take some deep breaths, and fall blissfully asleep.

How you wake up in the winter is equally as important as how you fall asleep. As you awaken, repeat a winter mantra like "warm, grounded, energized," and take several deep breaths. Bring your knees to your chest and hold them there for 30 seconds, then move from side to side, giving yourself a nice back massage and twist of the organs and spine. Hold the twist for 10 to 20 seconds on each side, to detox the organs and flex the spine. Straighten your legs and lift them up one at a time, then together, rotating your ankles clockwise, then counter-clockwise. Sit up in bed and put your arms straight out in front of you, then rotate your wrists clockwise and counterclockwise. Make a fist and extend your fingers several times. Lower your arms, shrug your shoulders, loosen your neck, and hop out of bed. These micromove-ments are essential to get the bodily fluids moving, which is crucial in this dry season. Overnight we have a long fast—sometimes 12 to 15 hours or even more—and the bodily fluids are diminished. Stretch-ing helps to hydrate the tissues, which is so important to get the lymph system moving, the tissues hydrated, and the mind focused.[1]

Breathe ....

The breath work to practice for the season is *nadi shodhana*, or alternate nostril breathing. The benefits of this easy-to-do *pranayama*—Sanskrit for "breath work"—are vast.[2] Practicing nadi shodhana is particularly balancing for Vata dosha as it is deeply grounding. But I also find this practice to be beneficial for Pitta dosha, as one must slow down to get the full benefit of it. Both Vata and Pitta tend to rush and push through things—meals, exercise, relationships, meetings. Nadi shodhana forces one to sit still and pay attention to each inhale and exhale, slowly and mindfully. Kapha dosha usually does not have a problem going slowly, so this breath work is a natural for them, and they will also benefit from the deep inhales and cleansing exhales. All doshas reap rewards from this in winter, as it warms with its gentle flow and is actually re-invigorating in that it highly oxygenates the blood.

By inhaling in one nostril and exhaling out the other, a mesmer-izing loop occurs, weaving together the chakras—our energy centers. It is said that inhaling on the right side sends the oxygen to the left side of the brain, and the exhale allows the flow to originate on the right side of the brain. In the ancient practices the great teachers noted that the left side of the brain, called the *pingala*, is the masculine (sun) side, and the right side of the brain, called the *ida*, is the feminine (lunar) side.

This pranayama actually balances both hemispheres of the brain, balancing our male and female tendencies. All that from breathing! No wonder this is the most revered form of pranayama, reportedly able to heal all maladies.

Nadi Shodhana
(Alternate Nostril Breathing)

Sit in a comfortable position on the floor (on a chair or a bed is fine, but make sure your chest is open and that you have room to raise your right arm with your elbow bent and at a right angle from the body). Sit straight. Place the tip of your tongue on the ridge behind your front teeth, called the Fire Point. This will reduce stress in the jaw and prevent clenching of the teeth.

With your right hand, close your index finger and middle finger into the palm, and keep the thumb, ring finger, and pinky extended. This is called Vishnu Mudra. Use your right thumb to gently close your right nostril and inhale deeply through the left nostril, expanding your belly like a balloon. Exhale fully through the same nostril keeping the thumb in place on the right, then inhale deeply again to the belly, and at the top of the inhale, close the left nostril with the right ring finger, open the thumb on the right, and exhale through the right nostril. At the end of the exhale, pause, then inhale deeply again through the right nostril, then close your right nostril with your thumb and exhale left. Then inhale left, close, and exhale right. Work up to 20 cycles (each inhale and exhale is one cycle), taking your time to increase. Begin with just 5 to 7 breaths on each side the first time, and slowly increase every time you sit down to practice.

As you breathe, visualize the life-force coursing through you, creating a stillness of the mind and body. This breathing practice creates deep rest and relaxation of the nervous system. Remember that it is in a body at rest that true healing takes place. With any pranayama, if you feel dizzy or out of breath, end the practice and resume normal breathing until you feel better.

Body Massage.....................................

A standard everyday practice, usually in the morning, is to anoint yourself with oil—lots of it! Beginning your morning with a warm oil massage starts the process of ridding the body of toxins that accumulated overnight, as well as igniting your own inner pharmacy.

I use an electric kettle in the bathroom to heat up water for drinking as well as for heating up my body oil. While the water is warming, this is a great time to start your oral routine. Look at your tongue and note the color and if there is any coating. A white coating indicates a Kapha imbalance, a buildup of ama—literally undigested food in your gut. A yellowish coating indicates a Pitta imbalance—too much hot, spicy food and ama. A dark, shadowy coating indicates a Vata imbalance—perhaps too many cold, raw foods and not enough lubrication. Use a tongue cleaner to scrape your tongue: beginning in the way back (it is said that gagging a bit can help to rid the body of toxins, but don't go too far back), use medium pressure and scrape forward 6 to 8 times, rinsing off the scraper in the sink after each scrape.

Then brush your teeth with a natural toothpaste. I like Auramere, Himalaya, Jason, and Desert Essence brands. You want to make sure there are no additives like fluoride, unnatural whiteners, or sodium lauryl sulfates in your toothpaste. If the tube says "do not swallow," then I say do not put it in your mouth! Gargle with sesame seed oil for 1 to 2 minutes to further rid the mouth of unwanted bacteria, as well as to leave a thin coating to protect against bacteria introduced during the day. Spit the oil into a trash can, not down your sink, or it can clog the pipes. Do all this before drinking anything so that you can wash out the unhealthy bacteria that accumulated overnight on the tongue, gums, and cheek tissues.

Now it's time for your massage!

This can feel especially luxurious in the late fall and winter as our joints, bones, and tissues are craving the extra lubrication and heat. *Abhyanga*, as the practice is called, penetrates the layers of our tissues, through the muscle, fat, nerves, blood, plasma, and bone, all the way to our reproductive tissues, nourishing each layer along the way. The massage action stimulates the lymph system, helping it to dump toxins out of the body, as well as stimulating your own healing power.

In winter use sesame seed oil or an herbal blend designed to reduce Vata dosha. Check in with yourself, though, to see what is needed. For instance, if you are more Pitta and run hot, try mixing coconut oil with sesame seed oil for your daily massage. Kapha and Vata can add a bit of mustard seed oil if feeling especially cold or lethargic.

Once the oil is warm (I let my bottle sit in a Pyrex cup of hot water for about 3 minutes, but you can also run the bottle under hot water), you can begin your massage. Using long, deep strokes, cover your body from head to toe with the oil, moving up and down over the long bones and in a circular motion over your joints. If you do not have time for a full-body massage, focus on massaging your joints, head, and feet. If you have the time, allow the oil to deeply penetrate the skin by leaving it on for 15 to 20 minutes before bathing.

After the massage, you should typically shower or bathe to remove excess oil. Leave a thin layer of oil on the skin to stay moisturized and to keep environmental toxins out—this includes your laundry detergent, fabric softeners, and dryer sheets, which can leave toxic residue on your clothes. That is why it is extremely important to use nontoxic, natural detergent and fabric softener and plant-based dryer sheets.

There are times, though, when a bath is not recommended. If you are experiencing any of the following, do not bathe (a quick shower will suffice): fever; gas or bloating; after a heavy meal; if you have diarrhea or loose stools.

Winter Essential Oils ....

Essential oils are particularly powerful in the winter months, bringing a sense of warmth and comfort to the body and at the same time invigorating and illuminating the mind. They also have medicinal qualities. Many oils are antibacterial and when you inhale, the nanoparticles enter the body through the nasal passages, making their way to your lungs and the limbic brain.[3]

These nanoparticles that enter the body can have a profound effect. The antibacterial qualities of some oils can begin a physical healing process, and just as important, the scent of the oils can begin an emotional healing process. Releasing emotions is essential to mental health, and smells are one way to gain access to memories—good and bad—allowing you to revel in the positive ones and release the negative ones. Certain scents can take you right back to a specific place and time, like how the smell of chalk can suddenly bring you back to elementary school and erasing the blackboard for your teacher. For me, the smell of Revlon lipstick reminds me of my mother, and Old Spice reminds me of my dad getting ready for work in the morning. Identify what scents make you feel good and what you would rather avoid. Take a few minutes to recall—or even meditate on—the root of the feeling that the scent awakened. If it is a negative thought, use your senses to visualize what occurred and how the scent came to be associated with it, and see if you can separate the two. Allow the reaction to the scent to become neutral, not related to the incident, so you will be less triggered by it in the future. If you have a happy or pleasant memory associated with a certain smell, it can be useful to also identify the connection to an experience, one that you can perhaps bring to mind to lift your spirits as needed. Keep that essential oil nearby so that you can use it whenever necessary.

In winter, you want to create feelings of grounding and warmth as you uplift the senses. Oils such as cinnamon, clove bud, fir needle, frankincense, myrrh, sage, sandalwood, sweet orange, vanilla, and vetiver are traditionally thought of as winter oils. One of my personal go-to blends for the season is eucalyptus, lavender, and tea tree oils. I mix it with unscented cream or oil and rub it on my chest at the first sign of a cold or sore throat. The blend is handy to use with a vaporizer or steam inhaler as well. It is very powerful, so a little goes a long way! See Remedies for Vata Season Ailments on page 66 for exact ratios. On a dark, cold morning when I am craving something to spark my spirit, I love using a blend of clove, bergamot, and cinnamon.

You can also easily create your own quintessential winter protection blend, commonly known as thieves oil. The story goes that there were four thieves who survived the Black Death (now known to be the bubonic plague) in the Middle Ages. These men robbed the dead yet never caught the deadly disease. Once they were captured, they revealed that they had avoided the plague by oiling their bodies with an essential oil mixture, which we now call thieves oil. Centuries later, we still use this blend for protection from illness! Here is how you can make your own.

THIEVES ESSENTIAL OIL

30 drops of lemon oil
20 drops of cinnamon bark oil
15 drops of clove oil
15 drops of eucalyptus oil
10 drops of rosemary oil

Combine the oils in a sterilized glass bottle with a dropper. (Use a 10- to 15ml amber or blue glass bottle to prevent light damage.) If you have sensitive skin, add a carrier oil (jojoba, almond, avocado) directly to the bottle, or you can mix your carrier oil and the thieves blend together in the palm of your hand (about 1 drop thieves to 4 drops carrier oil). Store in a dark, cool place. I keep mine next to my bed and rub it on my feet and neck, behind my ears, and on the top of my scalp every night before bed. You can also use this versatile mix as a household cleaner! It has amazing antibacterial and disinfecting qualities.[4]

How to Use Essential Oils
. . . .

While some essential oils can be used directly in their pure form, most oils need to be infused into a carrier oil. By mastering simple preparations such as scrubs, compresses, and diffusion, you can create a whole shelf of amazing products for a fraction of the cost of buying them already prepared.

It's very important to note, however, that you should never consume or orally apply essential oils unless a professional has given you the okay.[5] There are very few essential oils that can be ingested (with the exception of applying clove oil topically, which is an ancient remedy for sore gums and teeth), and unless you are a professional aromatherapist or working with one, I would avoid consuming them altogether.

It is always wise to test the blends on a small patch of skin first before applying them to your entire body. Do a scrub test on the inside of your forearm. If after a few hours everything looks good, then you can use the product on your whole body, avoiding sensitive areas like the genitals, around the eyes, and anywhere else you have sensitivities.

SALT OR SUGAR SCRUBS: So easy to make, you will want a dozen with different scents to keep all over the house! Keep a jar by the kitchen sink to help remove food smells like fish or garlic from your hands, one in the shower for full-body exfoliation, and one by the bathroom sink for a gentle face wash. Sugar is gentler on the skin, so you can use that for face scrubs. For hands and body, I prefer to use salt.

I recommend using an organic carrier oil like almond, olive, grapeseed, or jojoba, since these are more easily absorbed by your skin. Coconut oil is a great choice for summer or in warmer climates. You can add an unscented liquid soap to reduce the oily residue on your skin. For kitchen use, add

1 teaspoon of baking soda to help reduce odors. Grapefruit is amazing for the face. Chamomile and lavender for a calming evening bath or shower. Vetiver for a winter rubdown. Rosemary, sage, or peppermint is lovely for the kitchen. Adding a little honey to a face scrub is scrumptious!

To make your scrub, in a large bowl, whisk or stir together 1 cup sea salt or sugar (organic raw sugar is best), 1/2 cup carrier oil, 1/3 cup honey or 1/4 cup baking soda (if using), and 10 to 15 drops of essential oil. Mix well, then spoon into a jar with a tight-fitting lid. This will keep for up to 6 months. Just make sure to keep the lid tightly closed when not in use.

COMPRESS: A great way to use essential oils is to saturate a towel or washcloth with hot water and a few drops of oil. Allow the compress to cool slightly, then apply it to any part of the body where there are aches or pains, discomfort, or even rashes or hives. To make a compress, fill a small bowl with 2 to 3 cups hot water and 2 or 3 drops of a healing essential oil like ginger for sore muscles, or eucalyptus or peppermint for a headache, sinus problems, or congestion. Lemongrass or tea tree oil can treat fungal infections. Lavender is great for aches, pains, and bruises. Use chamomile for red, inflamed areas. Soak a washcloth in the mixture and press it to the affected area. Hold it there until it becomes cool, then soak it again. It's good to start with hot water in your bowl so you can keep applying the compress for 10 to 15 minutes.

INHALATION THERAPY: For coughs, colds, or upper respiratory infections, deeply inhaling certain oils may actually kill infections and open up the respiratory system. To make an effective remedy, heat up a pot of water—about 6 cups. Either pour it into a large bowl or use it directly from the pot. Add 1 to 2 drops each of lavender, eucalyptus, and tea tree oils. Drape a towel over your head, close your eyes, and lean over the bowl or pot, then inhale deeply though your nose, alternating with mouth breaths as well. This is a very powerful blend, so be sure to keep your eyes closed. Do this for a long as you can—5 minutes is great. The antibacterial and antifungal properties of these oils can help heal your ailments. You can do this 2 or 3 times a day.

Exercise..

A complete routine is always a combination of aerobic activity, stretching, and some weight or resistance training. Brisk walking, followed by stretching and some resistance work can be a full workout. In the colder months, working out in a gym or taking indoor classes can keep you motivated. Using at-home regimens like biking or rowing or yoga is also great—whatever works for you. Just keep moving!

Yoga is always a good idea, as it is a complete mind-body system of movement. By being aware of your breath and the movements of your body, you are being present and mindful. A good yoga teacher will encourage you to be present and focused on your movements and not to go too far—"no pain, no gain" does not apply in yoga! Yoga encourages you to go within, to find yourself in the pose, to explore and expand.

Try to find a yoga studio with no mirrors or music. Both of these take you away from your core reason for being there: to concentrate on yourself with little distraction. If you practice at home, set up a sacred space, ideally where you can see (or be in!) the outdoors. Yoga helps us to balance all five elements—space, air, fire, water, and earth—through precise movements aligned with your breath. It is the gateway to inner and outer harmony.

Hot yoga, however, should be avoided—or practiced with caution—as it can aggravate the doshas. I do not recommend hot yoga for any dosha, but especially not for Pitta. Even though Pittas *love* the heat and sense of challenge that comes along with it, it increases their fire to an unhealthy level. Hot yoga increases blood pressure and can cause dehydration, and it is no way even close to any classical form of yoga. Ayurveda does not believe in taking your body to extremes, which upsets our equilibrium. Suddenly introducing intense heat stresses out your body as it tries in vain to cool down. You are not detoxing in a hot yoga class. You are simply sweating out water and salt. Hot yoga is a Western invention that, in my opinion, has no place in a healthy daily routine.

Slow, strengthening yoga and exercise will gently warm the body and release stress and anxiety. Tai chi or beginner yoga classes will be greatly beneficial. If you find yourself feeling sluggish and putting on weight, you will want to follow a more physically intense workout, which should last for a slightly longer duration. Kapha should work up a good sweat, which will help shed those extra pounds, reduce ama in the system, and give you more energy.

Get Outside!

Kapha and Pitta can think about going outdoors and exercising in the fresh air in the colder months—a vigorous walk, cross-country skiing, or snowshoeing can be fun. Even a fast walk with the dogs (my favorite!) is highly beneficial to both you and the pups. Since people who are predominantly Vata dosha are typically cold, if you want to go outside to exercise just make sure you are bundled up and that you have a thermos with a warm drink with you.

In addition to getting some much-needed movement, getting outside gives you a chance to absorb vitamin D, which is key to staying well emotionally and physically, especially in winter. It's important to get sun on your limbs and torso whenever possible. Maybe some winter sunbathing? Between ten a.m. and two p.m., the sun is the highest (this is called the Pitta time of day). If it's not too cold out, roll up your sleeves and pant legs and go outside for 10 minutes or so.

In the morning and early evening, all doshas can do the ancient Ayurvedic practice of sun gazing. Using a *dristi* (slightly unfocused) gaze, look toward the sun and let your body fill up with vitamin D. You can also add these foods to your diet any time of year for a vitamin D boost: cod liver oil, salmon, swordfish, canned tuna, mushrooms, yogurt, eggs, milk, sardines, liver. There are now many studies showing that vitamin D can prevent cancer and other diseases.[6]

Studies show that the optimal times for exercise are from six to ten a.m. and six to ten p.m., so you can choose the time that best suits your lifestyle and daily routine. This time of day is related to Kapha dosha—the earth element. We tend to be a little sluggish during this time, so it's good to do the opposite—get moving. If you begin exercise just before six a.m., you will have the winds of Vata blowing, giving you a gentle push![7]

Meditation ....

Excess Vata is distracting and disturbing, sometimes increasing anxiety and worry, so practicing silent or guided meditation in Vata season is essential for your mental well-being. Our meditations in this season are aimed at helping us to be still, and this practice will help you to look at what is going on without engaging in it, allowing it to be present but not disturb you.

To begin, find a comfortable place to sit. In the morning, sit facing east, if you can—toward sunrise, taking in the natural energy of the day. In the evening, face north, a more relaxing, calming energy. You can sit on the floor, on cushions, or on a chair, sofa, or bed. If you need to, support your back with pillows or cushions, or sit on the edge of your chair or cushion. Your spine should be erect, but not rigid, shoulders down, chin slightly tucked. Relax your face, relax your body. Try sitting in an easy pose—cross-legged, or in half or full lotus position, but if this is uncomfortable, move your legs to a position that you can maintain for 5 to 30 minutes. You can place your hands in your lap or on your thighs, palms up or down, or in *chin mudra*—with the tip of the thumb gently touching the tip of the index finger—whatever is most comfortable and natural for you. Try to be free of distractions, or accept and make peace with your surroundings (like dogs or cats, city sounds, outside noise, etc.). Take 2 or 3 deep breaths to your belly and exhale fully, until there is no air left in the belly. If you have not eaten yet, do alternate nostril breathing (see page 52) to warm yourself up. Do not do this breath work on a full stomach. After 10 rounds, place your hand back in your lap and begin to breathe naturally.

Allow yourself to relax by watching the breath, noticing the slight rise and fall of the chest. Do not try to control your breathing—just notice. Bring your awareness to your solar plexus area, your belly, and above your navel. Allow the belly to be soft, no gripping, no holding. Feel the warmth in this area. You can even place your hands on your belly. Allow the warmth to radiate through your entire body. Feel it in the soles of your feet, your toes, moving up your calves, knees, and thighs. Sense your torso filled with warm light, your hands, fingers, and arms, notice the warmth move up your spine to your neck, your ears, to the crown of your head. Then bring it back to your belly.

Begin to silently repeat your personal mantra if you have one, or use *so hum*—which translates from Sanskrit to "I am the divine light within." Align *so* with your in-breath and *hum* with the out-breath. Feel yourself sink into the stillness of winter, when the earth rests. The fields are fallow. The trees are bare. Growth takes a break. Energy is reserved. Take shelter from the cold. Go within. Notice your thoughts, but do not engage in them. Just watch. Witness. Allow them to move by like clouds in the winter sky. Come back to your breath and the mantra over and over again.

Meditate for however long is comfortable for you, using a timer or an app. For beginners even 3 to 5 minutes is good. Try to work up to 20 to 30 minutes. At the end of the meditation, you can stop repeating your mantra, take a few deep breaths, and sit quietly for a few moments before opening your eyes. Open your eyes gently, looking downward, and slowly allow the gaze to move up. Wiggle your fingers and toes, stretch out a bit. Notice how you feel. Pay attention to the shift from meditation to a more waking state of being. Give thanks to yourself by placing your hands at prayer pose (*anjali mudra*) and bow deeply to honor yourself and your practice.

Practice to Tone the Root Chakra ....

Our subtle energy body also needs to be nourished and protected year-round. The chakras are our energy centers, and are thought to be connected to physical and mental well-being. Each of the seven main chakras, which are aligned with the spine, connect to deep-seated emotions related to our organs and glands. Since we crave home in winter, the root chakra (the first chakra, *muladhara* in Sanskrit) is our main focus. It keeps us grounded yet connected to all the upper chakras, sending deep roots into the earth, while at the same time reaching toward the light in the sky. Related to the earth element, the root chakra helps to balance the properties of space and air that are prevalent in winter.

Sit in a warm and comfortable place with little distraction. Use sandalwood, fir needle, cypress, or a seasonal scent like clove or cinnamon essential oil—1 drop of essential oil to 4 drops of carrier oil, or use a diffuser, or place a few drops on a tissue or cotton ball and inhale deeply. If using a carrier oil, rub the blend onto the soles of your feet and the palms of your hands. Make sure your body is at ease and that you are not feeling any pain or discomfort. If you are, adjust accordingly. Take a few deep breaths into the belly, gently close your eyes, and allow your awareness to move to the base of your spine, your sits bones, your perineum area. This is the seat of the root chakra. Imagine the entire area filling with a deep red light. This may begin as a small ball of energy, but allow it to grow in dimension until you feel or visualize the light filling your body. The root chakra is the equivalent of home, where our elemental needs are met—shelter and food, safety, security, survival. Use these words to stay focused on the root chakra:

FLEXIBILITY:
adaptability to outside forces

TRANSFORMATION:
awareness that problems can be
changed to creative opportunities

COHERENCE:
our unified purpose

STABILITY:
being in a state of centered
awareness even in uncertainty

Silently repeat each word slowly until just the very essence of the energies are left. As you sink deeper into the visualization and mantra repetition, you can begin to chant aloud (or silently, if you prefer) the sound *LAM* (*l-ahhh-m*). This is the sound of the root chakra. Chant *LAM* three times slowly, take another few minutes in silence, then open your eyes slowly. Place your hands at *anjali mudra* (prayer hands) at the center of your chest. Bow to yourself, your ancestors, and the winter season, which gives us permission to be still, grounded, stable, to go within.

When you finish your practice, you may want to have some hot water with ginger, or cinnamon and honey to warm the body.

Remedies for Vata Season Ailments.......

Winter is notorious as being cold and flu season—try as we might, we usually catch a little something. As we know, prevention is the first line of defense. Washing your hands, keeping your fingers away from your eyes, nose, and mouth, and not touching contaminated surfaces are some of the most important things you can do. If you do come down with something, these remedies should help.

COUGH AND COLD: Inhalation with essential oils (see the inhalation therapy recipe on page 59). Mix 1 tablespoon each of cinnamon and honey in a small bowl and lick it off a spoon 2 to 3 times a day. Drink licorice powder tea (you can also buy Throat Coat tea). Use nasya oil (oil for the nasal passages and sinuses) to lubricate your sinus passages and block unwanted environmental toxins; you can find nasya oil on Ayurvedic websites, or just use organic sesame seed oil.

SORE THROAT: Gargle with a mix of 1 teaspoon salt and 1 teaspoon ground turmeric in 6 ounces warm water. Lick manuka or raw, organic honey off a spoon. Drink ginger and lemon tea; add honey after the water has cooled off bit. Gargle with sesame seed oil.

DRY SKIN: Use ghee on particularly dry patches, after a warm bath or shower; or sauna, rinse, and apply sesame seed or coconut oil to damp skin, then, after 10 minutes, pat off any excess oil. Stay hydrated with warm fluids all day long; avoid excessive caffeine intake (it is a diuretic). If the skin is itchy, use calendula cream or neem oil.

DRY EYES: Bathe your eyes in ghee—fill swimming goggles with 1 to 2 tablespoons melted ghee, let it cool a bit, then fit the goggles over your eyes, lie down (with a towel under your head), and keep your eyes open and blinking for 5 to 10 minutes (this is called *netra basti* in Sanskrit); you can also fill an eyewash cup with ghee and hold it against each eye for 5 to 10 minutes. You will need to rest for at least a half hour after this treatment.

DRY SINUSES: Apply nasya oil morning, noon, and night. You can also use sesame seed oil, olive oil, or melted ghee in your nostrils. Just put a few drops on your pinkie and swirl around inside your nostrils. Do not use a neti pot in a dry climate or if you have dry sinuses.

DRY/CRACKED LIPS: Use a good lip balm that contains natural ingredients and oils; use nonpetroleum products like Alba Botanica Un-Petroleum Multi-Purpose Jelly. Stay hydrated. Avoid licking your lips.

CONSTIPATION: Take triphala tablets or powder before bed with your golden milk (see page 152); 2 to 3 tablespoons aloe vera juice three times a day; 1 tablespoon psyllium husk mixed into water in the morning or evening; or senna tea (try Smooth Move, Tulsi Lax, or Get Regular) just before bed. Take it for 7 to 10 days, but no more. Sip warm water throughout the day and eat lots of warm, sautéed, roasted, or stewed plant-based foods high in fiber.

JOINT STIFFNESS: Massage with heating oils like mustard seed, castor, or mahanarayan; Banyan Joint Balm and Maharishi Ayurveda Muscle Ease balm contain all the best ingredients. Exercise regularly—move it or lose it! If you have access to a hydrotherapy pool, try walking or working out in it a few times a week. Eat ghee; reduce cold and dry foods in your diet; and eliminate nightshades (tomatoes, peppers, eggplant), as they can increase inflammation in the joints.

WINTER COMES TO AN END

We begin to feel the changes after the winter solstice on December 21, as each day becomes longer. We know we are moving toward spring, a time of renewal. But don't rush through winter—allow yourself to feel the full benefits of slowing down, staying home more, nesting a bit. Soon the days will warm up and we will be making our way out of the cave for more vigorous activities. Kapha season begins in early spring. Enjoy the winter, find happiness by looking within. Allow yourself to do less and feel stress and anxiety melt away. Don't expect so much from yourself—you don't always have to be on alert! Winter gives us this gift. Receive it.

CHAPTER 4

Kapha Season (Spring)

KAPHA

. . . .

E arth and Water. Late winter through spring. Focus on detoxing, ridding the body and mind of accumulated, stagnant ama; lighten up, increase ojas, and reveal new growth.

• • •

QUALITIES:
damp, cool, heavy, soggy, sticky, and soft

ELEMENTS:
water and earth

DOSHAS MOST IMPACTED:
Kapha (wet, cold), Vata (change, cold)

TASTES TO FAVOR:
bitter, pungent, astringent

TASTES TO AVOID:
sweet, sour, salty

COMMON AILMENTS:
seasonal allergies, virus, flu, increased mucus,
congestion, asthma, common cold

DAILY BODY MASSAGE (ABHYANGA):
use invigorating strokes with sesame seed oil,
mustard seed oil, or sunflower oil blend;
dry brush; herbal powders

• • •

Spring has a tendency to sneak up on us. One day you're wearing a wool scarf and hat, and the next the sun feels warm on your skin and short sleeves are in order. Tiny sprouts make their way to the surface, getting ready to bloom as the sun's rays penetrate the soil. Heavy rains bring welcome relief to ground that became dry and cracked in the winter cold. The elements of spring penetrate our bodies, nourishing our tissues and warming our bones just as the earth is warmed and plants begin to grow. Along with renewed growth, the days begin to lengthen, the extra light lifting our moods and practically begging us to come outside and play.

In the Western Hemisphere, we begin to see the changes in the climate sometimes as early as mid-February and in some places as late as mid-April, and it is during this season that we begin to feel the qualities of Kapha dosha, which is composed primarily of water and earth. These elements are the attributes of spring: cool and damp with new rain or melted snow; slow growth, heavy soil, muddy earth, and a feeling of fullness. Early in the season we may feel dull, inert, bloated, and congested from increased mucus and sinus pressure. As the air warms up, the mucus will begin to drain and excess water will be absorbed by the earth, supporting new growth to unfurl, and we are rejuvenated.

When your Kapha dosha is in balance, the elements of water and earth come together to create stability and stamina—a foundation that holds the other doshas together. When Kapha is balanced, one rarely gets sick and is able to turn the natural caregiving qualities innate in Kapha toward helping others. But when Kapha is out of balance, the water and earth elements are out of control, creating a sticky, muddy mess—lethargy, stagnation, stuckness. At this point Kapha forgets to take care of themselves, withdraws, eats when not hungry, gains weight, and hides in their cave.

Ayurveda tells us to look for the opposite action in order to create balance. In Kapha season that means we want to lighten up. To beat back the cool and damp, we work to stay warm and dry; to combat the weight and slowness, we move more and cultivate new habits. As the plants, flowers, and buds begin to bloom, so do we. There's a reason we call it "spring cleaning"! This season is a natural time to clear away the debris to make way for new growth, and support detoxing of mind, body, and spirit.

Spring increases the qualities of Kapha dosha, so the rituals for the season are designed to reduce kaphic qualities. These rituals will help you lighten up and slough off the congestion and buildup of extra layers (ama and Kapha accumulation, i.e., weight) gained over the winter months. This is the ideal season for a detox cleanse—you'll find a protocol on page 80—and generally to focus on being more rigorous in your exercise, be more mindful of your hunger and appetite, and notice the seasonal shifts in circadian rhythms, adjusting your sleep time accordingly.

You may have put on a few pounds while in hibernation as our digestive fire—agni—is higher in winter, so we naturally eat more. Spring is nature's way of telling us to get moving and begin a steady march away from winter. The detox plan will rid the body of winter accumulation and excess ama, as well as seasonal allergies that may be creeping up on you.

As we align ourselves with the season, it's important to note that spring can be fickle, varying in temperature between cold and warm, wet and dry, windy and calm—a combination of all the doshas, which can make it difficult to settle into a consistent routine. It's crucial to be extra vigilant during this time and to implement rituals to keep us aligned in our bodies and support our overall health. I often find myself warmed by the morning sun and forget to bring a sweater or scarf when I leave the house. For this reason, I always keep an extra pullover and scarf in the car so I'm ready when the cool air catches up with me. The body uses a lot of energy to adjust from warm to cold and back again, and if we are not eating right and wearing the proper clothes (as well as moving, breathing, and sleeping well), our energy becomes depleted, and that is when disease can find a place of entry.

Ayurvedic wisdom says that disease occurs at the transition of the season for exactly this reason. And while I know it's only anecdotal evidence, the only time I ever get sick is when the seasons change! We need to be extra vigilant, and these are the times to be keenly prepared to practice our self-care rituals.

Allow yourself to flow with the changes of the season, and avoid being rigid and inflexible. Let the weather guide your day, your food and drink choices, your daily routine—and be prepared for whatever Mother Nature has in store.

Finding balance in Kapha season means focusing on detoxification—physical as much as mental and spiritual. All the rituals in this season are focused around giving your body space to capitalize on the natural urge toward regeneration and new growth in the spring. Spring offers the opportunity to not only clean out the leftovers from winter, but also to create new ground to build upon for the rest of the year. This season is key to preparing the foundation for the summer, fall, and winter. If we do well detoxing, scrubbing, and scraping out excess Kapha, we will have prepared our mind and body for the heat, dry, and cold of the rest of the year. This means we will be strong, healthy, sturdy, stable, and steady. Our roots took hold in late winter and now are branches reaching toward the sky, all on a solid foundation that will not fail.

During Kapha season, all doshas will benefit from focusing their diet on lighter, fresh foods, including bitter greens, heating spices, and drying and astringent ingredients. A liver cleanse is also critical in spring, since toxins have accumulated and compounded in our bodies during the winter months.

Mentally, our detox should reemphasize mindfulness and awareness. By implementing a mind-clearing meditation practice, we set ourselves up to refresh and renew for the season. The use of aromatherapy will fill your senses with invigorating floral, herbaceous essential oil blends to balance the mind dosha and bring you more into harmony with the season.

Our spring practices also include toning the heart and throat chakras, which offers a chance for the earthiness of spring to move up toward the air and space we need to balance the heavy energies of the season. Additionally, our self-massage practice moves away from warming oils to using powders or a dry brush to mitigate the sticky, thick, slimy qualities of the Kapha season. Along these lines, how we practice pranayama—breath work—this season is designed to activate the metabolic system, clear the mind, expand lung capacity, and strengthen the body to ward off seasonal ailments.

DINACHARYA FOR KAPHA SEASON

Eat ....

I can't think of a better time to take advantage of the season to change your diet and habits than spring. After the heavy meals of winter, spring offers us an opportunity to reduce the amount of food we consume daily, as the body no longer needs to convert those calories to heat us up and aid in digesting the substantial food (and larger portions!) we were drawn to during the winter. In spring, nature provides us with the exact ingredients we need to pare down again while feeling satisfied

In spring, all doshas can benefit from eating less.[1] Not only is fasting (for some) an important tool for detoxing, but eating less has been proven to increase longevity and to decrease cardiovascular disease.[2] What an incredible gift for those needing to lose weight! Unless you have a severe Vata imbalance and have difficulty keeping weight on (if that is you, eat seeds and nuts or sweet fruits between meals as needed!), allow the digestive system to rest between meals, avoid raw, hard-to-digest foods, and keep the quantity small. When you fast between meals, the body is forced to use stored energy (what you accumulated over the winter) to keep going. This is how we detox—getting rid of those stored pockets of ama (undigested food).

No matter your weight loss goals, significant benefits can be found in eating the fresh, light, and nutrient-dense foods widely available in spring. Emphasize the tastes of bitter, pungent, and astringent in your diet and greatly reduce sweet, sour, and salty. Also try to avoid all dairy, wheat, and sugar. When I lost 60 pounds in my early Ayurveda days, it was because I stopped eating all dairy, wheat, and sugar. The weight dropped off—as did 80 points off my cholesterol! Over time I was able to reintegrate foods like bread and the occasional sweet or ice cream back into my diet—but I am keenly aware when it's gotten out of control, and I try to avoid these foods altogether in spring.

Apply your "spring cleaning" urges to your pantry and fridge, and eliminate foods such as milk, cream, yogurt, ice cream, aged cheese, pasta, breads, chips, tomatoes, sweet citrus fruits, nuts, and red meat. I would even add alternative plant-based "meat" here like Beyond Meat and Impossible Burgers, as the manufactured proteins they are made of are heavy, oily, and clogging. These are considered sweet, sour, and salty foods (densely nutritive). Lessen your intake of these foods during this season.

Go-to springtime foods include a variety of bitter greens like dandelion greens, mustard, mizuna, arugula, radicchio, endive, and rapini (broccoli rabe). You will want to lightly sauté the greens or add them to soups and stews. And go crazy with cilantro and parsley—adding them to just about anything savory you are eating, including the occasional egg, beans, fish, and chicken—as they will help all your food become more Kapha-reducing.

Other bitter, pungent, and astringent foods include hot peppers, ginger, cloves, thyme and basil, yellow and green veggies, lentils and other legumes, beans, seeds, pomegranates, black tea, and cranberries. Look for tart cherries, unripened bananas, green apples, and other sour fruits to satisfy cravings. You can find a complete list of Kapha-appropriate foods on page 135.

And, of course, don't forget the spices! Known for their medicinal qualities, spices have been revered and valued for thousands of years for specific healing purposes as well as great taste.[3] Specifically in spring, we all benefit from using more ginger, black pepper, coriander, turmeric, cinnamon, cloves, and cardamom. I love the Spring Spice Churna below and use it as my go-to blend all season long. I make a batch and store it with my spices to use for kitchari, rice, and lentil recipes and even on eggs and in soups. This way all my seasonal spices are in one jar and I don't have to go on a hunt through the spice cabinet every time I cook. Additionally, I make a small container to carry with me to add to food when eating out, as most restaurants—unless they are ethnic—use pretty bland "spices" or rely on just salt and pepper. This blend can even help to lighten up foods that are heavy for the season like avocado toast and potatoes. Totally yummy.

SPRING SPICE CHURNA

1 tablespoon ground ginger
1 tablespoon freshly ground black pepper
1 tablespoon ground coriander
1 tablespoon ground turmeric
1 teaspoon Himalayan salt
1 tablespoon ground cinnamon
Pinch of cayenne pepper

Combine all the spices in a small glass jar or stainless-steel container with a lid. Seal the container well. Store in a cool, dark place for up to 1 year. You can use this at home for cooking or take it with you when you eat out. It will not only make your food taste more delicious, but it will help to balance Kapha dosha in the spring or any time Kapha needs reducing.

As always, drinking warm water with lemon (lime for Pitta) is beneficial to all doshas. Citrus contains compounds called hesperidin and flavonoids, which scientific studies have proven to have protective qualities for the liver. Among their many biological activities, flavonoids present in lemons and limes have radical antioxidant and anti-inflammatory properties.[4] Drinking lemon or lime water in the morning also helps to alkalize the body by reducing acids that have accumulated overnight.

Often when I suggest to my clients that they begin their day with hot water and lemon or lime, they say that someone in their family used to do that, usually their mother or grandmother. It's an ancient tradition in so many cultures—make sure it becomes one of your traditions, too. I usually have a large glass of warm water with either lemon or lime by my side throughout the day. My favorite kitchen gadget is my citrus squeezer.

I also recommend a spring tea made from herbs that contain pungent, bitter, and astringent qualities. Drinking 1 to 2 cups each day will help to reduce congestion, stuffiness, and lethargy we can feel in springtime. You can try my Spring Tea (page 78 or 155), or choose from the herbs and spices on page 78 to make your own! (Ready-made blends are okay, too, in a pinch.) Sipping the tea throughout the day is also a great way to keep these cleansing herbs coursing through the body, doing their work to detox, clean, and rebuild the tissues.

SPRING HERBS AND SPICES

Ginger

Peppermint

Tulsi

Clove

Cinnamon

Cardamom

Turmeric

Cayenne pepper

Cumin

Fennel

Black pepper

Licorice

Fenugreek

SPRING TEA

Try the "other" CCF (cumin, coriander, fennel) tea for spring.

2 green cardamom pods

1/2 teaspoon coriander seeds

1/2 teaspoon fennel seeds

Steep the pods and seeds in 3 cups just-boiled water. Strain the tea into a mug and sip throughout the day. You can add more hot water as needed. I use the same seeds for 3 or 4 cups of tea. *Optional:* If you have spring allergies, add 1/2 teaspoon stinging nettles to the mix, or drink stinging nettle tea on its own during the allergy season.

Honey is one of your best friends this season, as raw, organic honey can actually scrape excess Kapha from the body. Remember, though, that you should never cook honey or add it to very hot liquids, as high temperatures can kill off its healing qualities. Allow tea to cool off a bit before adding honey.

Remember that spring is cool, heavy, and wet so we want to do the opposite to mitigate those kaphic qualities. Look for food that will wring out the excess Kapha we accumulated in the winter—foods that will dry, warm, and lighten the system.

Support Your Liver

The liver is the washing machine of the body. Anything we can do to boost liver function, especially in spring, is welcome. That includes cutting back on alcohol, sugar, unnecessary dietary supplements, and oily, fried, and fatty foods—anything that taxes the liver should be avoided. Try to buy only organic food, if you can, as conventionally grown or raised foods may contain pesticides and herbicides, which may contribute to fatty liver disease.[5]

Two Ayurvedic herbs that are superb for cleaning the liver are *bhumyamalki* and *manjistha*. These two herbs are readily available and are usually included in herbal blends for liver cleanses. You can purchase them in powder form to mix with warm water, or as tablets. These are especially helpful at moving sludge out of the liver (and the gallbladder as a bonus!), as they are super bitter. It's difficult to find this level of bitter in our food, so taking these supplements can be very helpful if you feel you need a boost.

If you live in India or near an Indian market, however, you may be able to find some extraordinarily bitter foods. Karela, also known as bitter gourd, is an amazing cucumber-like vegetable that is extremely bitter and, honestly, a little hard to eat. But cooked with oil and salt, it can be quite refreshing! And if you can find amla, aka Indian gooseberry, stock up for spring, as it will also promote and strengthen liver function.

Modified Kitchari Cleanse
• • • • • • • • • • •

Many Ayurvedic sites recommend doing a spring cleanse with kitchari. This Indian comfort food is an easy-to-digest vegetarian stew made with split yellow mung beans, basmati rice, spices, and vegetables. While I think this is great, I have come to prefer this recipe made with whole green mung beans, which I first had while undergoing panchakarma, the Ayurvedic detox and cleanse, in South India. My husband and I were on a 21-day cleanse and ate this kitchari every morning. You would think we would get sick of it, but once we got back home, we continued to eat it nearly every morning! For a cleanse, eat just this for 3 days, for breakfast, lunch, and dinner. Make sure to drink plenty of fluids throughout the day including Spring Tea (page 78 or 155), ginger tea, or just hot water with lemon or lime. You can add honey to your tea (just wait until it has cooled a bit before adding the honey).

VAIDYAGRAMA GREEN MUNG DAL CLEANSE

SERVES 2

1/2 cup dried whole or split green mung beans
    (moong dal; if whole, soak overnight or for at least 6 hours,
    then drain and rinse)

3 to 6 fresh curry leaves (you can buy fresh and freeze)

1/2 teaspoon ground cumin

1/2 teaspoon ground coriander

1/2 teaspoon ground turmeric

1/2 teaspoon ground ginger (optional)

Pinch of hing (asafœtida)

1 heaping tablespoon coconut oil or ghee

2 carrots or 2 celery stalks, chopped (optional)

1/2 to 1 teaspoon salt

Leafy greens, like dandelion greens, mustard greens, or spinach
  (optional, but great for you)

Optional garnishes: unsweetened shredded coconut, raw unsalted
  pumpkin seeds (can dry roast in a sauté pan), fresh cilantro or
  parsley, squeeze of lime juice

Place the mung beans in a large soup pot and add 2 to 4
cups water. If you start with just 2 cups water, you can
add more if you want it to be soupier. Bring to a boil over
medium-high heat, then reduce the heat to maintain a simmer. Add the curry leaves, cumin, coriander, turmeric, ginger
(if using), hing, and coconut oil or ghee. Cook for about
20 minutes, until the mung beans are soft. If you are using
carrots or celery, add them after about 10 minutes.

Taste and season with salt. Ladle into bowls and add
whichever garnishes you like. Serve hot. This kitchari is ideal
for breakfast but can be enjoyed anytime, and is also delicious
served over white basmati rice.

Sleep...

Ah, Kapha and sleep—they go together like cookies and milk! Kapha
loves her deep, long slumber and tends to sleep through just about
anything. Even if you are not primarily Kapha dosha, you, too, may be
seduced by the heavy qualities of spring and sleeping in. As the days
become longer, there is an urge to stay up later, but try to keep your
bedtime consistent at around ten or eleven p.m. In every season, but
especially in spring, you will benefit from sleeping during that crucial
period from ten p.m. to two a.m., when Pitta dosha is highest and

your digestive fires heat up. Nutrients are assimilated into the tissues and waste is readied for elimination in the morning, and the increase in agni will help you to break down everything that you ingested over the course of the day. And I don't just mean food: thoughts, images, and emotions need to be digested as well. So it is imperative that you allow your body to go through this natural cleansing process every evening. If not, you will accumulate ama (toxic residue) and won't feel your best.

On the flip side, you'll also want to resist the Kapha urge to sleep late. Wake with the sun when possible! The sun begins to rise earlier in the spring, and you can use those extra hours of daylight to amplify your energy and creativity. Kapha time of morning is six to ten a.m. You may naturally awaken at the end of Vata time (two to six a.m.), but the temptation to turn over and catch a few more winks can be compelling. But notice that when you wake up in Kapha time, you probably feel a bit foggy and lethargic. Think back to your feeling when you woke up at five thirty—you were probably wide awake, right? So it's up to you—another hour or so just to wake up groggy, or hop out of bed during Vata time and use that motivation for meditation and your daily routine? You decide!

It is especially important to avoid napping, as sleeping in the daytime increases Kapha—the opposite of what we want to accomplish. If you are elderly, pregnant or lactating, a young child, or ill (either mentally or physically) and must nap, try to keep it to 20 minutes. Any longer than that, and you will wake up with that heavy, sticky, sluggish Kapha feeling.

Vata types are light sleepers and often struggle with insomnia because the excess space and air in their dosha can create an overactive mind. Ever wonder where the term "second wind" comes from? Vata dosha staying up too late! If people with a Vata imbalance wake up between two and six a.m. (Vata time of night), it can be very difficult for them to get back to sleep. If this happens to you, resist turning on the light or looking at your phone. Instead, practice vagus nerve relaxing breath (see page 48), repeat a soothing mantra such "deep sleep" or chant the root chakra mantra *LAM*, or sit up and meditate for 20 minutes. Then try going back to sleep.

Pittas are typically sound sleepers, though they tend to sleep for shorter periods of time. But even competitive, sharp Pitta will benefit from 8 hours of sleep, if possible. Best to get that sleep on the early side of the night to take advantage of the ten-p.m.-to-two-a.m. timeframe. Pitta usually does, however, feel refreshed even with less sleep. So you be the judge, but don't criticize yourself (as Pitta is wont to do) if you feel you need a bit more shut-eye. Do you need an alarm to wake up, or do you wake naturally? Do you wake up hungry or hangry? Do you feel cool or overheated? Ask yourself these questions so you can be your own practitioner and decide what is best for you. (Hint: Hangry probably means you overslept, as Pitta is usually hungry when they wake up. Ditto for overheated.)

Exercise...

The extra hours of daylight are a gift to get you moving and breathing. Walking outside is one of the very best ways to align yourself with the season and to feel great. Fresh air, sun, the sounds of nature and animals balance the system naturally. Kick off your shoes and "earth"[6] a bit—10 to 20 minutes of bare feet on the earth each day can help you sleep better and reduce stress and anxiety.

Whether or not you can get outside, cardio is the name of the game during this season. An ideal routine would include 20 minutes of aerobic activity like walking, jogging, rowing, or riding a bike to get your heart pumping and break a sweat—both of which help flush toxins from your body. You can follow this with a period of stretching and flexing, concentrating on your limbs—including ankles, shoulders, fingers, and toes. Neck circles, extension of arms overhead with a slightly arched back, then hands to the floor and a few twists will keep the blood flowing and help the lymph to get rid of toxins. Then spend about 10 minutes working with weights, using hand weights or machines at the gym. It's always a good idea to check in with a trainer, if you have one available, to create a plan for you.

All doshas will benefit from the toxin-removing action of per-spiring. Try to work up a sweat in whatever exercise you choose. If you are primarily Kapha dosha, go for the full sweat. Kapha is a cold dosha, and you need to generate a lot of heat to detox. Vata dosha should feel the workout heat up gently in their bodies, slowly moving from the bones to be muscles to the skin as your body warms. When you feel like you have completed a good workout, stop, rest, and recover. Vata tends to work out to depletion and exhaustion, taxing themselves so much that they crash for hours in order to regain their strength and energy. Pitta, be aware of overexertion and pull back when you feel out of breath or are sweating profusely—this is an indication that you have gone too far. While Pitta loves to challenge themselves (and others), a balanced Pitta knows when they have had enough and can let go of the competitive edge. Slow down and allow the body time to cool down.

The ideal time to exercise for all is during Kapha time, from six to ten a.m. Second best time is Kapha time in the evening, six to ten p.m., but if you choose to exercise later in the evening, notice how it affects your sleep. It's not always right for people to work out close to bedtime, and if you find that you're feeling revved up or too hungry, maybe it's better to consider adjusting your routine.

Note that it is better to meditate *before* exercising, as it can be hard to settle back down after vigorous movement. I do, however, always recommend doing some light stretching or a sun salutation (or seven—one for each layer of the tissues) before settling down to meditate.

Exercise for Your Dosha

· · · · · · · · · · ·

You will also want to make some adjustments for your own specific dosha type. For example, if you're a hot, intense person—whether you are a true Pitta or just having a Pitta moment—you will want to go to the extreme, only to quit when your routine becomes unattainable. Be patient with yourself, and try to rein in the impulse to go all out—more is not always better! Slow down and feel the incremental achievements as you work on your routine. The best exercise for Pitta in the spring is walking, light hiking, or noncompetitive bike riding. Swimming is also great for Pitta. Keep the timing to 20 to 30 minutes and focus on relaxing into the movement.

Vata dosha will do best with gentle yoga, tai chi, or swimming in warm water. Vata does enjoy running but that causes extra air and space in this already spacey dosha, so keep faster-paced activities to a minimum. Use lighter weights and more reps for your workout. This will help to increase strength without overtaxing you.

Kapha dosha benefits the most from increased movement in springtime. Exercising to produce a sweat is ideal. Fast walking, biking, or light jogging are all good activities, but avoid the pool—remember, like attracts like, and being in the water amplifies the watery elements of Kapha. Better to move on dry land.

I used to swim—a lot. It was my go-to exercise for years, and I couldn't imagine why I still weighed over 220 pounds. I would glide through the water and feel so light for a mile or two, then sit on the side of the pool and drink a bottle of water. I never lost a pound. Swimming also increased my appetite and, as I learned later, increased my Kapha. When I was discovering Ayurveda, I read a book called *Ayurvedic Healing*

Cuisine by venerated teacher Harish Johari. He said those with a Kapha imbalance should not drink so much water. I was stunned. I always thought drinking copious amounts of water was healthy! But Johari, in all his great wisdom, clued me in to this notion of like attracting like.

Once I moved out of the pool and began sweating it out in the gym, drinking less water, and following my ideal Ayurvedic routine, the weight literally fell off. Who knew?! Well, Ayurveda did! And now you do, too.

Breathe ....

Because it works on both the body and the mind, our breath is one of our most powerful tools of alignment and self-regulation. In spring, we want to focus on breath work that clears the mind, increases awareness, and sharpens the senses. Kapalabhati Pranayama (Skull Shining Breath) is an ideal practice for spring, as it increases energy, removes excess mucus from the lungs and nasal passages, and makes the mind shine! In this practice, the inhale is passive and the exhale is forced, which helps to clear the paths in mind and body, creating a lightness of spirit mentally and physically. By creating movement within the body and stimulating synovial fluid to flow, you will prepare the body for a super-clear meditation practice.

Kapalabhati is also a natural choice for ridding the body of stagnation and increasing circulation. However, for this reason, please note that it is contraindicated if you are: pregnant; have high blood pressure, glaucoma or serious eye issues, or migraines; have had a stroke; or have recently had a C-section or abdominal surgery.

Kapalabhati Pranayama
(Skull Shining Breath)
• • • • • • • • • • •

Sit on the floor with your hips slightly elevated, with crossed legs, or sit on the edge of a chair. Close your eyes and begin breathing in and out through your nose, taking several deep breaths to your belly. Once you've found your rhythm, begin to forcefully expel the breath through the nostrils, pulling your belly button toward your spine as you exhale. Allow the belly to expand slightly as the inhalation happens passively, effortlessly. Then immediately begin another forceful exhalation, same as above. Try to do 15 to 20 rounds, ending on an exhale in which you completely empty your lungs. Sit quietly and allow the breath to return to normal. Slowly increasing the rounds will build resiliency, increase metabolism, and strengthen lung capacity. If you'd like, do another round. You can slowly build up the practice by increasing the number of rounds to 30, 40, 50, and eventually to 100 breaths. If you feel unsteady or dizzy, stop immediately, allow your breath to return to normal, and rest.

This practice is best done in the morning on an empty stomach. If you have eaten, you will feel nauseous, as you are increasing pressure on the abdomen. If you find yourself feeling low-energy at other times of the day, feel free to do the practice, but wait until at least 2 hours after eating.

Meditation ....
There are as many meditation practices as there are people. Each individual comes to meditation with their own unique makeup, circumstances, expectations, and challenges. Much like balancing the doshas, we can curate our own best practices for meditation, and over time you'll find what feels most comfortable to you. For ex-

ample, some people prefer to sit cross-legged on the floor on a zafu (meditation cushion), while others do better seated in a chair with their feet firmly planted on the ground.

All doshas will do well to stretch or take 3 or 4 belly breaths to ground themselves before beginning their practice. Using a timer can also help to settle the mind—you don't need to worry about the time or be distracted by watching a clock. Set your meditation app or use the clock function on your phone for however long you can dedicate to the practice. Then leave the phone by your side (facedown—those notifications can wait!) and let it watch the time for you.

You may also want to keep a meditation journal, noting the date, duration of the meditation, and emotions or any thoughts that surfaced that you'd like to return to. No need to write copious amounts—just a few notes can help you notice trends and challenges. When we see them on the page, we more easily find solutions.

Meditation is often best practiced in the morning on an empty stomach, but not every dosha will be able to concentrate. Pitta wakes up hungry and Vata may feel spacey, so it could be beneficial to have a small bite before your practice. Choose food that is low in sugar and definitely not processed. A good choice would be a handful of nuts for Vata or seeds for Pitta. Some fresh cheese (never aged) or paneer can also settle the stomach. Even a cup of herbal tea can satisfy hunger. Remember, though, that if you are going to include breath work, you will want to do that on an empty stomach. Since most pranayama practices take just a few minutes, you should be able to accomplish it before eating. Kapha dosha, on the other hand, usually does not feel hungry in the morning and can easily meditate on an empty stomach.

Rejuvenating your meditation practice in Kapha season will bring you a chance to do some much-needed mental spring cleaning! In your practice think about investigating the dusty corners of your mind, the overstuffed drawers, those closets filled with stories or beliefs that no longer serve you. Imagine shining a flashlight into those nooks and crannies, revealing negative thoughts, unwanted emotions, things you haven't dealt with in years. What have you swept into a corner and forgotten about? Stuffed under the bed or in the back of drawer? Now is the time to shine the light, reveal it, unpack the baggage, and sift through what is there. Take your time to look around at what you can throw away, get rid of what no longer serves you, make room for new growth, ideas, new potential.

Difficult emotions can be worked through by calling them forth to examine during your meditation practice. Be curious, and gently guide your attention to whatever you have been hiding, avoiding, or stuffing down. Simply put, look for what no longer serves you and resolve to let it go. You may find that after working with a negative emotion or situation, it is helpful to allow your thoughts to flow to a more positive feeling and let them fill the space. Alternatively, you may find peace by just leaving the space empty, but filled with potential for what may come.

End your practice with a resolution to let go of what is no longer needed. Mentally wrap it up in a box and offer it to the Universe. Feel the space you have created around you, and resist the temptation to fill it up right away. Rather, revel in the space. It is a place of potentiality. You will know when it's time to fill it up again.

As you end your meditation, you may want to make a few notes in your meditation journal about what you have resolved to let go of and what you may be interested in allowing into the space. Write it down and put it away. Let the Universe take care of it for you.

Chakra Toning..................................

Water and earth are the elements that predominate in spring and in Kapha dosha. This correlates to the root (*muladhara*) and sacral (*svadhisthana*) chakras, earth and water elements respectively. These two lowest chakras (near the base of the spine) will be especially active during this season. These chakras echo the attributes of spring—damp, earthy, grounded. However, to balance those energies and ensure that all chakras are aligned, we need to focus on connecting to two of the chakras: the heart (*anahata*) and throat (*vishuddha*). Connecting to these upper chakras can help you lighten up from the heaviness of earthy, wet spring, shedding winter stagnation and accumulation. Along the way we will encounter the heat of the solar plexus chakra, which will warm the air for our journey. The higher chakras—the third eye and the crown chakra—will complete the toning session, assuring that we are connected to universal consciousness and balancing with the elements.

What Are Chakras, and Why Do We Need to Balance Them?
· · · · · · · · · · · · · · · · ·

Chakra toning through visualization and meditation is a way to open circulatory channels in the body and increase the flow of energy. The more energy that flows through the chakras, the healthier we are. When the system is out of balance, the blocked energy is said to cause illness. Barbara Brennan, an energy healer and author, says that these blockages "also distort our perceptions and dampen our feelings and thus interfere with a smooth experience of full life."[7] Once we learn how to balance our chakras, we can begin to see our full potential as each chakra correlates to different emotions, organs, energy centers, elements, even colors, scents, gemstones, and sounds.

According to the ancient Vedic and Yogic texts, there are seven major chakras in the body, located along the length of the spinal column and connected to glands and subglands. This is called the *sushumna*. These centers of energy help us function on a subtle level, as well as emotional and physical levels. *Chakra* literally means "wheel" in Sanskrit. For reference, my favorite books are *The Chakras* by C. W. Leadbeater (written in 1927!) and *Llewellyn's Complete Book of Chakras* by Cyndi Dale.

To align your chakras in spring, begin by sitting cross-legged on the ground, or on a meditation cushion if possible, or in a chair, with the spine straight and chin slightly tucked. Bring your awareness to the base of your spine, where your body meets the earth. Imagine roots connecting you to the ground, to your home, a feeling of safety and security. The earth is moist and accepting, with warmth seeping in as the days grow longer and the sun shines brighter. Allow yourself to feel connected, accepted, and welcomed. Sit in that space as you visualize the color red filling the root chakra region. Allow natural urges and desires to arise while feeling connected to the earth, safe, secure. Chant aloud or silently *"lam, lam, lam"* (the "a" sound is like "ahh") and rest in the resonance.

Next shift your attention to the pelvic region—this is the seat of the sacral chakra. See if you can notice a sense of creativity, a sense of your unique sexuality. This is the fluid, water element. The sacral chakra offers a sense of being comfortable in your body, in your sacred abode. Visualize the color orange in the entire pelvic area and chant the sound *"vam, vam, vam"* (vaahm) and rest in the resonance.

Then allow your attention to move up to the navel region, recognizing the solar plexus chakra with the color yellow. The fire in the belly will help melt away the chill of winter. Feel your innate power to make your dreams come true. Chant the sound *"ram, ram, ram"* (raahm). Continue up to the center of your chest to the heart chakra, where the air element rules. The air lightens the heaviness of the season. Compassion, love, and forgiveness for self and others reside here. Know that the attributes of the heart chakra are infinite and unconditional. You can give and receive an endless amount of love, compassion, and forgiveness, and you need nothing in return to sustain you. Giving is the sustainer. Receiving unexpected love, compassion, and forgiveness is a gift. The color is the green of new growth. The sounds is "*yam, yam, yam*" (yaahm).

And now allow your focus to settle at the base of the throat, the vishuddha, or throat chakra. Feel your breath move in and out, from the cool air entering the nose, following it down the back of your throat and filling your lungs. The sense of air and space is located in the throat chakra, which includes your ears. Connect to speaking your truth as well as hearing the truth, and discerning what information is important for you hear. The color to visualize is blue. The sound is "*hum, hum, hum.*" Rest in the resonance.

Notice the difference, if you can, of the heavy earthiness of the root and sacral chakras, and the space-filled lightness of the throat chakra. Stay with the air and space. Allow yourself to feel light and airy, floating in the blue sky. After a few minutes here, allow your attention to scan the third-eye chakra—indigo with the tone of "*sham, sham, sham*" (sh-AAH-m)—and the crown chakra, violet with the sound of the Universe, "*om.*" Feel yourself rise above the body to the etheric realm and allow that lightness to fill your being, to counterbalance the qualities of spring.

When you are ready, slowly move back down through the chakras, visualizing the colors and hearing the tones, and come to rest in a still body. Notice again the cool air of the breath in the throat. Remember this feeling as you slowly open your eyes and enter into the spring season with lightness and ease.

Body Massage......................................

Oil can feel very heavy this time of year—or any time of year when you are having a kaphic imbalance, like weight gain, congestion, or feeling dull and lethargic—so pick up the dry brush for an excellent detoxifying technique. For dry brushing, use an all-natural bristled brush and stroke upward on your legs, torso, arms, chest, neck, and back, 8 to 10 strokes for each body part, toward your heart. This will increase blood circulation, exfoliate the skin, stimulate the lymphatic system, and invigorate you.

If you have skin issues such as eczema, hives, skin allergies, or psoriasis, you should not dry brush. Stick with oil. Vata dosha, too, will usually benefit more from the grounding benefits of oil, provided they are not feeling too stagnant.

Another great choice for body massage in Kapha season is *udvartana* or *garshana*. These massages use powder, paste, or raw silk gloves rather than a brush to increase circulation of blood and lymph.

GARSHANA GLOVES: These are massage mitts made from raw silk. The friction of rubbing the gloves on your skin will increase circulation of blood and lymph, which helps to detox the body and will create a beautiful, healthy glow to your complexion. Massage clean, dry skin (no oil) the same way you would using a dry brush.

UDVARTANA: Applying dry powder or a powder paste on the skin before bathing can help with weight loss and removing the accumulated effects of Kapha season. *Ruksha udvartana* is rubbing the skin with chickpea powder and ground ginger. You can add a little bit of sesame seed oil or water to make a paste, if preferred. This can make a bit of a mess, so be sure to stand on a towel or sit on a low stool in the bathtub or shower! You might also consider wearing a face mask to avoid breathing in the powder. Use upward strokes to cover the entire body and vigorously rub the skin. The benefits of this massage are vast—it improves circulation, reduces cellulite, increase weight loss, removes body odor, and increases mobility and energy.

You can make your own powder by combining 2 cups dried chickpeas and ½ cup ground ginger in a blender and blending until the chickpeas are ground to a powder. Extra powder can be stored in an airtight jar for up to 6 months.

After your massage, rinse off in the shower using a chemical-free body wash or soap (see below).

How to Wash After Abhyanga or Udvartana
· ·

We know that soap can have so many different ingredients—not all of them good for our skin! Commercially produced soap may contain chemicals for foaming, artificial dyes, and unnatural scents. Look for all-natural soap such as soaps made with essential oils, coconut, castile oil, or shea butter—Dr. Bronner's, Kirk's Natural Original, and Nubian Heritage are some of my favorites—or make your own! While I understand the desire to scrub the skin after treatments—or any time you take a shower—please keep in mind that your skin has a microbiome just like your gut. We need those beneficial bacteria on our skin to stay healthy and prevent environmental toxins from penetrating the dermal layer.[8] I like to tell my clients to rinse off (even without soap) and wash more thoroughly in "high traffic" areas—the groin, under the breasts, the armpits, and the feet.

When you do wash, one of the best ways, according to Ayurveda, is to use green mung bean powder. In India, after one is oiled or powdered, the panchakarma therapist washes you off using ground mung powder made into a paste with warm water—no soap! (Mung beans, aka moong dal, are usually available at most grocery stores in the Indian or Asian sections, and in Indian grocers and online; grind the dried beans into a powder using a blender or coffee grinder.) This mixture is rubbed onto the skin and poured over the head to remove just enough excess oil to leave a thin layer on the skin and scalp to continue nourishing the tissues. You can do this at home! A totally natural way to rinse without removing too much of your natural healing bacteria and leaving you smelling clean and fresh. This is a great Kapha season routine.

Remedies for Kapha Season Ailments.....

The increase of mucus and phlegm and uncertainty of the climate seem to contribute to a great number of ailments in springtime. As pollen increases in late spring, allergies that were dormant in the winter begin to resurge. Coughs, colds, flus, and viruses can run rampant in schools, offices, and the community. If you do become infected, Ayurveda has you covered.

In addition to the herbs and foods listed on page 135, getting enough rest is key. Stay home from work or other activities if you feel ill. Wash your hands and face after coming into contact with infected people. Don't exercise or push yourself too hard. There is an Ayurvedic saying: "You cannot fix an engine when it is running." You are the engine. You must stop running in order to heal yourself. Please remember this!

Here is a list of some common ailments and remedies that should keep you in the best of health during the season.

SEASONAL ALLERGIES: Quercetin in combination with stinging nettle will address the allergens directly rather than just the symptoms. You can take both as capsules or tablets, and drink 2 to 3 cups nettle tea every day during the season.

VIRUS AND FLULIKE SYMPTOMS: Stay hydrated by drinking tulsi tea. Tulsi reduces flu symptoms, and will also help to relax the nervous system, which creates a better environment for healing. Take ashwagandha tablets or powder (about 500mg) after eating; add plenty of turmeric to your food or drink ginger turmeric tea to reduce inflammation. Make sure to get plenty of rest and practice breathing exercises.

INCREASED MUCUS AND CONGESTION: Licorice tea will melt excess mucus. Dissolve 1/2 teaspoon licorice powder in hot water, or buy a prepared tea like Yogi Tea Breathe Easy. Drink 2 to 3 cups a day. You can also make tea with cinnamon, black pepper, ginger, and turmeric or add these spices to your food or soup. Honey also helps to scrape excess Kapha from the system. You can eat a few tablespoons a day or add honey to warm water or tea.

ASTHMA: Licorice tea will open the lungs and reduce inflammation, and it removes excess mucus and phlegm from the body; daily pranayama is a must. Practice alternate nostril breathing and, if you can handle it, Kapalabhati Pranayama (page 87). An added bonus of licorice is that it aids in digestion by lubricating membranes and facilitating healthy elimination.

COMMON COUGH AND COLD SYMPTOMS: The Ayurvedic herbs *sitopaladi* and *talisadi* will help remove excess doshas from the lungs and sinuses. They can also reduce fever. These come in powder form, which you can make into a tea or mix with a little bit of honey and lick off the spoon; if you have a stuffy nose and sore throat, mix 1 heaping tablespoon each cinnamon and honey in a small dish and lick this off the spoon. If you have ground pippali—long pepper—you can add that to the mix; eat this 2 or 3 times a day. Make a gargle with 1 teaspoon salt and 1 teaspoon turmeric dissolved in warm water and gargle with this mixture 2 or 3 times a day. Gargle every morning with sesame seed oil to soothe the throat and fight infection.

SPRING COMES TO AN END
CLEARS THE PATH FOR SUMMER

As spring comes to a close, I hope you will feel lighter, filled with energy, and excited about the possibilities summer has in store. If you have followed spring guidelines you undoubtedly feel clear, creative, and confident about the future. Kapalabhati Pranayama, meditation, and chakra toning offered gifts of renewal and rejuvenation, while spring foods nourished your mind, body, and soul. Sleep patterns changed from winter to spring, enlivening and nourishing you deep down through all the layers of your tissues, naturally facilitating a cleanse. As we began to move our bodies more—hopefully outdoors—we find ourselves in closer touch with nature and the elements. This creates the most profound sense of balance, nudging each dosha closer to their home, ridding the body of excesses that can cause illness and disease and boosting the immune system to be more resilient. Every component of our daily routine is designed with this in mind—eat, sleep, breathe, move, meditate—all to align with the season. To work with nature and not against it.

As the weather changes where you live, bring with you the results of the spring cleanse, which opened the path for the rich warmth of the summer and the gifts the wet or dry heat has to offer.

CHAPTER 5

Pitta Season (Summer)

PITTA
· · · ·

Fire and Water. June through September in most places in the Northern Hemisphere. Any time the temperature is consistently above 75°F. Focus on cooling the body by eating less and gravitating toward cooling herbs, spices, and foods. Heat can reduce appetite, so two meals a day may suffice, depending on your health and activity level. The long days increase outdoor time and shorten the sleep cycle.

·   ·   ·

QUALITIES:
hot, intense, pungent, light,
sharp, moist (humid), dry (arid), acidic

ELEMENTS:
fire and water

DOSHAS MOST IMPACTED:
Pitta, mildly Vata (dry heat and late summer/early fall)

TASTES TO FAVOR:
sweet, bitter, astringent

TASTES TO AVOID:
salty, sour, pungent

COMMON AILMENTS:
dehydration, heartburn, heat rash, heatstroke,
headache, hives, bug bites, sunburn

DAILY BODY MASSAGE (ABHYANGA):
use light, slow strokes with room-temperature coconut, sesame seed, or sunflower oil

•   •   •

The summer months can be full of activity, vacations, and, for some, kids home from school. There is a general sense of being more carefree, of timelessness and ease that is so different from the rest of the year. Sometimes there may be an increased level of activity that ultimately can leave us feeling lazy and lethargic due to the heat. To acclimate to the warmer weather, we wear lighter, less constricting clothing, which can lead to a feeling of being freer, perhaps even open to more possibilities. The urge to kick off our sandals and walk in the grass is powerful. And just like in winter when we long to connect to the earth—maybe by making a snow angel—in the summer we long to lie on our back and watch the clouds move by or sit on the beach and listen to the ocean waves crashing on the shore.

While it may be hot outside, be aware of the varying temperatures when you enter office buildings, shopping malls, supermarkets, or theaters. The air conditioning in those places can be frigid, so always be prepared with an extra layer. And even though it may be cold inside, there is no fooling our body that it is hot outside, so you will want to keep the practices outlined here in mind even if you work in a cold office building or as you dash in and out of the car, stores, and businesses. You still need to follow the guidelines for the summer season and keep the self-care rituals aligned with the natural world—not the "unnatural" world of man-made climate control.

The qualities of Pitta dosha can be seen and felt on a typical summer day. In the mid-Atlantic region where I live, the seemingly contrasting qualities of hot and wet (humid) make up the weather from late May to late September. Those same contrasting qualities—fire and water—are the elemental makeup of Pitta dosha in Ayurveda. How can fire and water coexist? The humidity in the air and the water in Pitta help to balance heat and fire. They are actually complementary to each other. Without the water element, Pitta heat would damage the tissues and organs of the body. Hot days without humidity can spark devastating wild fires with tragic consequences as we have seen over the years in dry places. This is why we balance with opposite actions.

Without adequate balance, Pitta will just explode, leaving a trail of scarred, scorched earth and people behind. So keep in mind the stabilizing qualities to keep Pitta in check. Remember, Pitta is hot, sharp, penetrating, spreading, intense. Aim to be cool, less demanding, and perfectionistic; contain your thoughts and feelings that are critical or judgmental, and relax—just chill out!

You may sleep less due to the heat, which is natural. But strive for comfort using a fan or air conditioning set to a coolish temperature—cool enough for you to feel comfortable, but not unnaturally cold. Notice your appetite and eat accordingly. We are usually less hungry in summer, so if you are not hungry, try not to eat just because the clock says it is a mealtime. Look closely at the summer self-care rituals, which are designed to take heat away from the body and mind through meditation, breath work, exercise, and the food we eat.

Summer daily rituals should leave you feeling refreshed and re-invigorated, ready for the day. Whether physically or mentally, adjusting your practices for the Pitta season will allow the seeds you planted in the spring to grow and flourish.

Summer is literally ripe with yummy food choices—from mint juleps and summer designer drinks, to eating juicy red watermelon, grilling outside, and hearing the music of the ice cream truck slowly making its way through the neighborhood. From soft and sweet peaches and plums to succulent mangoes and luscious melons, summer is abundant with wet, sticky, and sweet fruits, just in time to beat the heat. The joy of the season spills over into its food and many of the natural choices are light and cooling. We simply don't crave as much food in the hot months as our digestive fires (agni) are naturally on a low simmer in order to keep the body temperature cool. Heavy food becomes harder to digest as energy is diverted away from the digestive process and stomach acids are reduced. The hotter it gets outside, the lower your agni, and decreasing digestive powers result in a naturally reduced appetite. Pitta season is a great time of year to allow the digestive system to take a break—maybe eating just two meals a day if that works for you. Less fat, and more raw or lightly cooked foods. Juicing for one of those meals is a great way to get a nutritional boost without creating extra heat needed to digest fibrous food.

While the heat of summer tempers our digestive fire, it has the opposite effect on our emotional fires: scorching days can make us irritable, angry, frustrated, even downright mean! We know from the description of Pitta dosha that when overheated and out of balance, Pitta can be quite damaging to themselves and others. At the same time, the Pitta sense of competition and rising to the challenge can lead to destructive consequences. Even if your primary dosha is Vata or Kapha, the hot, long, dry, or humid summer days can sometimes bring out the worst in all of us. If you are feeling overly critical, judgmental, aggressive, angry, mad, or hot-under-the-collar, look for ways to cool down emotionally as well as physically. If these situations arise, drink some cool mint tea or coconut water. Have some melon, a cucumber salad, or even ice cream or sorbet (it's hard to be mad when you are eating ice cream!). Take a cool shower or a swim. Don't, however, take a run in the noonday sun, eat a spicy burrito, or have a Bloody Mary. Watch your reactions, and be vigilant about your breath work, meditation, and chakra toning to bring as much cooling as you can to your emotional landscape.

If you are lucky, you may just have some extra time on your hands to use to increase the duration and frequency of your meditation. Taking pleasure in the time you have to offer to your practice can really reap rewards down the line. A morning and evening meditation of 20 to 30 minutes is ideal, allowing the cooler temperatures of dawn and dusk to infuse your practice with calming, restorative energy. Try facing east in the morning to capture the essence of the rising sun, and north in the evening to take in the cool lunar energy. As you will see in the meditation section for summer (page 116), you can be light and easy with your practice, in an effortless method.

As summer winds down, we enter into the early fall season, even before the temperature decreases. During the dry and light qualities of the late summer days we begin an accumulation of Vata dosha, which becomes exacerbated and aggravated as we venture deeper into fall.[1] This is the time of year to begin adding more lubricating foods into the diet, such as increasing fats and starches, and reducing the cooling carbs and raw foods we ate all summer long.

The Power of Color

Pitta-soothing colors are greens, blues, purples, white, pearl, cream, pale yellow, and light gray. This color palette will keep you cool mentally and physically. It also helps to cool down the people around you. Wearing fiery red, bright orange, or sunshine yellow will increase the heat people see and that you feel.

I once had a client who was a very high-achieving Pitta. She insisted on wearing power red to work nearly every day. She was an executive and had several people working under her. Tall and blazing with Pitta's fire and intensity, she ran a tight ship and was very successful at her job. She was also a loving, caring, sweet person, but when her coworkers and staff saw her coming, they would scatter in fear of the Red Warrior. She truly wanted more connection with her people but could not get through to them on a deeper level. I suggested she begin to wear Pitta-pacifying colors like cool blues and light greens. She embraced the idea, and immediately things changed at work. Staff began coming around to talk with her. People were no longer wary of her and began to share more in meetings. She was invited to lunch by folks who had never done so before.

The power of color! Remember that the next time you wonder how you can change dynamics in your workplace, at home, and in your relationships. Something as simple as changing the color of your clothes can change everything.

DINACHARYA FOR PITTA SEASON

Eat ....

Keep it cool, light, and less—my motto for summer eating!

As always, we want to eat to balance the natural qualities of the season—so it is best to avoid foods that heat up the system in hot weather, such as raw onions and garlic, tomatoes, yogurt, citrus fruits, and alcohol. Luckily, nature offers a bounty of easily digestible and cooling foods all summer long. To stay nourished, lean more toward foods that are sweet, bitter, and pungent. Melons, berries, cherries, coconuts, cilantro, mint, and an abundance of cooling sweet fruits and fresh and detoxifying greens are perfect this time of year—and all in season! White meat and fish are okay, but steer clear of red meat. Lighter fats such as ghee and coconut oil should be your go-to for cooking.

If you stick to your seasonal offerings, you will be rewarded with excellent digestion as your gut microbiome naturally adjusts to the food available locally. Remember, even though your local store may have everything on the shelves, from root vegetables to hot sauce, stick to the Pitta seasonal shopping list (page 138), or better yet, visit your local farmers' market and choose locally grown foods. Be aware, though, that many farmers still spray their crops with pesticides and herbicides, so unless the farmer specifies it, "local" does not mean organic. Seek out organic farmers to support them, and your health. The gut microbiome needs the local food, but it does not need glyphosate,[2] the active ingredient in the herbicide Roundup, which has been linked to fatty liver disease, cancer, and other illnesses.[3] Choosing locally grown, easy-to-digest foods will keep your digestive system running at the low speed it is designed for in summer.

You may think you need to forgo using spices in the heat of summer. While I wouldn't recommend adding too many chile peppers, there are some spices and ingredients that are perfect antidotes to the season. In Indian restaurants, yogurt-based raita (often with cucumber) is usually served with spicy foods, as it will help to cool down your mouth and tummy. Spices like cumin, fennel, peppermint, coriander, and cardamom are actually cooling! Flavorful salts and the Summer Spice Churna (see below) are simple additions to any meal and help to balance summer heat while keeping your food flavorful, healthy, and satisfying.

SUMMER SPICE CHURNA

Handful of crushed fresh or dried mint leaves

2 tablespoons coriander seeds

2 tablespoons cumin seeds

2 tablespoons fennel seeds

1 tablespoon green cardamom seeds

1 tablespoon ground turmeric

1 teaspoon ground cinnamon

1 teaspoon ground ginger

1 teaspoon coconut palm sugar, Sucanat, or jaggery

1/2 teaspoon sea salt

Combine all the ingredients in a spice grinder or blender and grind to a powder. Transfer to a glass jar or other airtight container. Store in a cool, dark place for up to 1 year. Add to any savory foods. Fill a small container to take with you when you eat out.

FLORAL SUMMER SALT BLEND

My dear friend Michele Schulz, an Ayurvedic chef, educator, and yoga instructor in France, created this brilliant and simple recipe for summer salt. Use this beautiful rose-pink salt any time you are having Pitta imbalance as well as throughout the heat of summer.

In a blender, combine equal amounts of mineral salt, dried organic rose petals, and dried hibiscus flowers and pulse until the rose petals and hibiscus are powdered. The resulting salt will be a deep shade of pink. Store in a saltshaker and use as needed in place of table salt, at home and when you eat out.

There is a very interesting concept in Ayurveda about the taste and effect of food in the mouth, called *virya*, and postdigestive action, called *vipaka*. For example, we avoid raw onions and garlic in summer because they are hot and pungent in that form. But once they are cooked, they become sweet and actually Pitta pacifying. So the postdigestive effect of cooked onions and garlic is sweet—enjoy these delicious offerings cooked in the summer, and raw, if you like, or lightly cooked, in the winter.

Healthy and Not-So-Healthy Food Combinations

In Ayurveda, foods don't just have flavors, but also specific tastes (sweet, sour salty, bitter, pungent, and astringent) and postdigestive energies (cooling, heating, light, heavy, lubricating, drying). When food is combined properly—like beans and rice, a pairing found in nearly every culture—we are able to easily assimilate the nutrients and effectively get rid of waste. The food digests smoothly without negative side effects like gas and bloating. But when we mix together foods that are incompatible, the results can be damaging to our system and result in indigestion, fermentation, gas, bloating, altering the microbiome, allergic reactions, and even setting the scene for illness and disease. Food is medicine, but just like any prescription, you have to get the dosage right to nourish the body and mind, prevent disease, and increase longevity. In a similar vein, there are many food combinations that we would consider "contraindicated."

The science and theories behind the combinations can seem complicated, but the goal is to ensure that your digestive process isn't working at cross purposes, and that the food you eat digests at the same rate. For example, in Ayurveda we say to eat fruit on an empty stomach, either 45 minutes before a meal or 2 hours after a meal. Why? Fruit digests at a faster rate than most foods, so when mixed together, the fruit will digest first, creating a fermentation process in which the rest of the food will "stew" until you are able to produce more stomach acids to break it down. To avoid this, eat fruit on its own and allow it to digest properly. I suggest eating a bowl of berries, a slice of melon, or seasonally appropriate fruit in the morning before your main meal. It should stimulate your appetite and you will easily absorb its phytochemicals and nutrients.

OTHER RULES INCLUDE[4]:

- Avoid mixing milk with bananas, cherries, sour fruits, melon, yeasty bread, meat, yogurt, beans, and rice.
- Don't eat the same amount of honey (heating) and ghee (cooling) together.
- Avoid eating raw and cooked foods together.
- No beans with cheese, fruit, milk, yogurt, or meat.
- Eggs should not be combined with milk, yogurt, cheese, or melon.
- Avoid hot drinks when eating yogurt, meat, fish, or cheese.
- Don't mix lemons with cucumbers, milk, tomatoes, or yogurt.
- Melons should always be consumed on their own.
- Eat one protein source per meal.

This season you should also think about the manner in which you prepare the food as well as the temperature of the food. Not to spoil your summer cooking, but why would you want to heat up your food and your surroundings when it's already so hot outside? Grilling in particular—despite being a universally popular summertime activity—is actually detrimental to your health and can create toxic chemicals in your food. Nearly all food cooked at high heat will produce acrylamide, a known carcinogen. You will also find acrylamide in any food processed at high heat, like potato chips and french fries. It is also found in cigarette smoke.[5] Be aware that any time you crisp or deeply brown your food, you are increasing the amount of this toxin.

Remember that Ayurveda is a science of opposites. Cool down your cooking techniques in summer to help create balance. Traditional Ayurvedic practice isn't crazy about smoothies because they are cold and, like we talked about, some ingredient combinations can be harmful to digestion and limit absorption of nutrients. However, I know that many of my clients swear by their morning smoothie, so I have found a way to work with that—Ayurveda wants to meet you where you are! With a few adjustments, you can create healthy, nourishing concoctions that are also delicious. You will find several creative ideas in the Seasonal Recipes section starting on page 141, but this smoothie is a personal favorite to beat the humid Baltimore summer.

SUSAN'S SUMMER SMOOTHIE

In spring when blueberries, raspberries, and blackberries are abundant, I freeze bags and bags of them. Again—Ayurveda does not love freezing food, but frozen organic fruits and vegetables can sometimes be more nutrient-dense than something that has been trucked across the country, or from another country and then sat in a warehouse for days before it made its way out to the produce section. If you can't find organic local produce, I think using frozen organic—which is flash frozen very close to where it was harvested—is a fine choice. If using frozen berries for this smoothie, thaw them in hot water for a few minutes, then drain, before using.

My smoothie is quite simple, with few ingredients. Often the simpler, the better! The chia and flaxseeds, in addition to adding essential omega-3s, will thicken the drink.

SERVES 1
1 cup fresh berries
1 tablespoon Udo's Oil, coconut oil, or flaxseed oil
1 tablespoon chia seeds
1 cup almond milk, warmed
1/4 cup canned full-fat coconut milk
Warm water, as needed

Combine all the ingredients in a blender or Nutribullet and whir it up for 30 seconds or so, then pour into a glass. That's it! Simply delicious.

If you are feeling heavy, hot, stagnant, or have a Pitta dosha imbalance, try taking aloe vera juice in the morning. This plant-based extract is nourishing to the tissues and extremely effective at removing excess Pitta accumulation from the liver and intestines, creating an internal "cooling" system in summer. Take about 3 tablespoons in the morning on an empty stomach.

There are other ways to stay hydrated and feel cooler in summer than just by drinking more. Some great, innovative ideas include adding hydrators like coconut oil and butter to your coffee (just a teaspoon each); adding chia seeds to soup, salads, and smoothies; eating quince, kiwi, pineapple, berries, sprouts, zucchini, radishes, romaine, and cucumbers[6]; and sipping water all day long to stay consistently hydrated.

Another counterintuitive but effective strategy is to keep drinking hot tea! Back in the day I lived in Tel Aviv, Israel, close to the beach. I would watch in bewilderment as people poured steaming-hot coffee and tea from thermoses into cups and sipped it in the sun. In like 100°F weather! There must be something to it, because I do find it refreshing to sip a mug of warm water with lime or warm (not really steaming hot) tea even on a hot summer day. There is comfort and groundedness to be found in holding your favorite mug.

The blend on page 112 is bound to cool down your system and delight your taste buds. If you like your tea a bit sweet, try adding an Indian sugar called jaggery, which is dried sugar cane juice. You can also try Sucanat (a brand name, derived from the words "sugarcane natural") or coconut palm sugar. Avoid honey in summer, as its metabolic process will create excess heat.

COOLING TEA BLEND

You can double or triple this recipe and sip the tea throughout the day.

SERVES 1 OR 2

1/2 teaspoon licorice powder
Pinch of ground ginger, or 1/2 teaspoon crushed fresh ginger
Pinch of ground cinnamon
1 green cardamom pod, crushed, or pinch of ground cardamom
Small handful of dried organic rose petals
  (optional, but delicious!)

Combine all the ingredients in a teapot or other container with a strainer, then pour in 1½ cups boiling water. Steep for 5 minutes, then pour through a strainer and enjoy.

Sleep...

In any season, Pitta is naturally highest from ten p.m. to two a.m., when the digestive system heats up to metabolize food, thoughts, and emotions—and often right when we're trying to sleep! The effects of these processes are even more amplified during Pitta season, so it's little wonder that it can be difficult to fall asleep when it's hot outside. Still, getting enough rest is essential to allow the body and mind time to restore and rejuvenate, absorb everything you took in during the day, assimilate the nutrients, and prepare waste for elimination, so in Pitta season we do all we can to cool ourselves down and calm our heated minds as we prepare for sleep.

Adjusting for longer days and increased sunlight is an essential first ritual in this season. As the sun sets later in the evening and rises earlier in the morning, the days get longer and longer as we approach the longest day of the year, June 21, and some areas may get anywhere from 13 hours to even 24 hours of light! If you are sensitive to light (Pitta dosha, in particular, can have light sensitivities), use darkening shades in your bedroom or wear eye shades. Try to be asleep by ten p.m., as Pitta time of night is revving up to high gear. By falling asleep around or before ten p.m., you can still get some of the lingering cooling benefits from Kapha time of night (six to ten p.m.).

If you do not live an air-conditioned home, using a ceiling or standing fan can really help. If you are lucky enough to live in an area where the air is cooler at night, definitely open a window. Sleeping naked can also help the body adjust to excess heat by regulating temperature. I also recommend using bedding that is light and cool. Trade out the heavy comforter for a light blanket and 100 percent organic cotton sheets. Some people miss the weight of a comforter, so you can look for "weighted" blankets that are still cooling.

There are also plenty of triggers throughout the day that can greatly disturb sleep in the summer including eating heavy, fried, or processed food for dinner or, worse, after dinner; not taking sufficient breaks during the day, especially to rest the eyes; or intense physical activity late in the day, which creates excess heat in the body and mind. All these actions will catch up with you when it's bedtime. So it is imperative to take the entire day into account when you look for reasons why you may not be sleeping well.

To get quality sleep in Pitta season, we have to focus on cooling not just the body, but the mind. Vata types have a chatty mind, whereas Pitta types will ruminate on unfinished business. Kapha is lucky to have fewer sleep problems. Take time before bed to do breath work or meditate, both of which help to calm the nervous system and can prepare both body and mind for sleep. You'll find a cooling breath work practice on page 115, and a suggested summer meditation practice on page 116.

A nighttime mini massage is also a great way to unwind. A self-massage of the feet and scalp with coconut oil or bhringraj oil can deeply relax your nervous system and induce a deep, restful sleep. Add a drop or two of rose, neroli, or sandalwood oil to enhance the benefits. You can even use the rose oil on your forehead and around your ears and belly button to add a cooling and calming sensation.

Sex is an often overlooked trigger, but especially in the summer, sex before bed can create aggravating heat and disrupt sleep patterns. Maintain moderation in sexual activity in the summer months and aim for the six to ten a.m. or six to ten p.m. time period. This is Kapha time—a bit cooler and slower. Take your time!

If you still notice yourself struggling to fall asleep, I recommend several winding-down techniques. Before bed, try sipping a warm or cool cup of mint tea or CCF with cardamom tea (1/4 teaspoon each of cumin, coriander, and fennel seeds with a pinch of cardamom steeped for a few minutes in about 12 ounces of hot water).

Avoid screen time in bed, as the blue light emitted by devices like tablets and smartphones messes with your circadian rhythms, blocking the production of the sleep chemical melatonin. I have some clients who swear by amber-colored glasses.[7] Amber is a cooling color, and wearing the glasses in the evening may allow the brain to release more melatonin to help you get to sleep.[8] Especially if you are looking at screens all day and again in the evening, amber glasses can mitigate the effects of mind-altering blue light.

When you do get ready to fall asleep, Ayurveda recommends sleeping on your right side in summer. It is said that the cool lunar energy enters through the left nostril, which can be cooling and calming for the mind and body. But if your tummy is full, sleep on your left side to aid digestion.

If you struggle with waking up during the night, you can sit up and turn on a dim light. This will help to shift your mind away from the agitation felt by being woken up or not being able to get to sleep. Keep a journal or notebook at your bedside so you can make notes of things that might be keeping your mind alert. Write it down and get it out of your mind and onto the page. You can also try reading something not very stimulating—maybe a spiritual text, a magazine article, or a passage from a book (but not on your phone or iPad unless you have night mode turned on).

Breathe ....

Sheetali pranayama means "cooling breath." People with an abundance of Pitta dosha should practice this all year, but all doshas can reap the rewards in summer, as this practice helps release excess heat from the body—and the mind! As with all breath work, practice on an empty stomach. This particular practice is great to do during the Pitta time of day, ten a.m. to two p.m. and before bed around ten p.m.

Note: This practice is done with a rolled tongue. If you cannot roll your tongue, follow the instructions for shitkari breath on page 116.

1. Sit in a cool, quiet location, if possible. Make sure you are seated comfortably either on the floor, on a zafu, in a chair, or on the bed. Let your spine be long but not rigid. Relax your shoulders. Slightly tuck your chin. Relax your belly. Close your eyes gently and take a few deep breaths with your hands either in your lap or resting on your thighs.

2. Stick your tongue out and begin by inhaling—slow and deep—through a rolled (like a straw) tongue. Then retract your tongue, close your mouth, and exhale fully through the nose. On the exhale, bring the tip of the tongue to the roof of the mouth on the ridge behind your front teeth. Repeat.

3. Work up to 5 minutes. In the beginning you may only be able to do a minute or so. Take your time to work up to a full practice.

If you can't roll your tongue, try shikari breath:

1. Make an exaggerated grin with your lips wide and inhale through the sides of the cheeks and your teeth, with your tongue flat and resting on the roof of your mouth behind the front teeth.
2. Close and relax your mouth and exhale through your nose. Repeat.
3. One to 2 minutes to start with is great. Work up to 5 minutes, or until you feel cooled down and refreshed.

End the practice by sitting quietly for a few minutes and feel the cooling sensation in the back of your throat and the warmer air leaving the body on the exhale.

Meditate ....

Take your time in your summer meditation. Even though for some people, summer revs up with lots of activities, it is actually the slow-down season. Allow the body and mind to pause, maybe even to be a little bit lazy. Meditation is all about being still—embrace those languid days! Allow the mind to move slowly from one thought to another without trying to stop it; just observe it. Sit back, relax, and watch the movie of the mind unfold without much interruption or interpretation. This is a mindful meditation designed to allow you to witness the comings and goings of your thoughts without trying to change them, grasp on to them, or cling to old patterns. View them as separate from yourself. Your thoughts and emotions are not who you are—they are just a collection of your experiences. By watching dispassionately, you can begin to let them go. As we begin the process of witnessing, we also let go of the idea that we have control. Control creates heat, the opposite of our summer plan. Sitting back, disconnecting, and watching the workings of your own mind without judgment or criticism will help you wind down and understand yourself at a deeper level. Watch for patterns that will help you get off the cushion (when you are not meditating). Hopefully you will begin to trust your intuition and follow your own inner guidance system.

Summer Meditation Practice
· · · · · · · · · · · ·

Set your timer for 20 minutes. Sit comfortably with your spine straight. Gently close your eyes. Take note of how your body is positioned, where your body makes contact with the chair, ground, cushion, or bed. Feel those contact points and relax yourself into them. Take some cooling sheetali breaths or alternate nostril breathing and sit back and watch the show. No need to control the thoughts or push them away. Take the opportunity to watch, listen, and feel; and let go, over and over again. You may find yourself sinking deeper into a state of no thought—don't resist—allow your mind to go where it needs to go. Watch. Witness. Stay present. No effort. Stay awake.

After 20 minutes, gently open your eyes, take a deep breath, and exhale fully. Stretch out your body and allow the meditation to integrate itself into your bones before rising up. Nice and easy. Take a few more deep breaths and bow deeply to yourself. Sip some water or tea and begin your day if you are meditating in the morning, or wind down for bed if it is evening.

Chakra Toning.....................................

The solar plexus chakra (*manipura*), just above the navel, is the power center. Pitta dosha is situated in this area of the body, the center of digestion, metabolism, and transformation. It is also said that our ego resides here. We hold on to people, power, and possessions in this chakra. When balanced we feel confident, assertive, and secure; when out of balance we are either materialistic, greedy, power-hungry, and controlling, or scared, distrusting, and suspicious.

The element associated with the solar plexus chakra is fire. The color is yellow. The sound is *"ram,"* like "r-ahh-m." Harnessing the power of this chakra can help you transform your life, relationships, health, and wealth. This is the chakra of manifestation, desire, intention, will, and destiny.[9]

To activate and balance this chakra, find a place to sit where you can see or be in nature. Try sitting in the cool shade or next to a body of water. The sound of wind chimes, flowing water, birds, or rustling leaves can bring you to a state of complete and total awareness. Take in your surroundings with all of your senses, then gently close your eyes.

Bring you attention to the manipura chakra, above the navel and below the breastbone. Place your hands on your belly and take several deep breaths, feeling your hands move as your belly expands and contracts. Then place your hands on your lap or thighs, palms facing up. Allow the breath to become natural. Feel the vibration in the belly and imagine, if you can, a turning wheel of yellow energy in the center of your torso. Notice the coloring, the shading, the intensity, the temperature. Is it a big wheel or a small one? Is it turning easily, or is it bumpy and inconsistent? Is it hot or warm? Just notice without trying to change anything.

As your attention stays on this area, begin to silently repeat the mantra of connection to this power center: Desire. Intention. Will. Destiny.

These are not goals; rather they are evolutionary suggestions that can be activated through practice. By stating your desires, your intention, your will, and your destiny, you will begin the process of spontaneously creating your reality, furthering your connection to your life's purpose. You don't have to have the answers, just use the mantra to awaken the impulses.

After a few minutes of repeating the mantra, slip into silence. Follow your breath and the sounds and sensations around you as you sit silently, integrating the practice, for another 5 to 10 minutes.

At the end of the meditation, place your hands in anjali mudra (prayer hands) and bow deeply to yourself and your surroundings. Feel a cooling sensation in your belly and know that any time you feel overheated, attached, greedy, or controlling, you can tap into your innate desires and let go of outside material forces.

Chanting Mantras

Science is beginning to study the truly fascinating effects that chanting mantras has on the brain. One study found that "neurophysiological correlates of religious chanting are likely different from those of meditation and prayer, and would possibly induce distinctive psychotherapeutic effects."[10] Another noted that chanting may therefore enable a beneficial lifestyle for health and play a role in the prevention of chronic diseases.[11] The Vedas say that repetition of certain sounds can calm the doshas. To balance Vata, we use the mantra *hrim*, which is pronounced with a hard "h," sounding like *khreem*. Pitta dosha can chant *aim*, pronounced like "I'm." Kapha can repeat *kleem*. The shape of the mouth and placement of the tongue can help to balance the doshas as you repeat these mantras out loud. Visualizing and repeating them silently also has a huge beneficial effect. Try using these mantras when you find you have a busy mind, trouble concentrating, or at the beginning of your meditation. I often use a mantra when I'm walking the dogs—much to their amusement—if I find my mind drifting into places where it does not need to go (like old issues, negative emotions, or just plans and lists). Repeating the mantra helps to take me out of that space and into the present moment where everything is usually fine.

Body Massage.....................................

If it is too hot and humid in your region to do a body massage with oil, I suggest using a dry brush instead. Still, you may want to just give it try with coconut oil at least once. It may sound counterintuitive, but you may be surprised by the cooling benefits. For a summer massage we use room-temperature oil rather than warm. In addition to coconut, sesame seed and sunflower oils are good, light alternatives.

This technique is traditionally performed before bathing. Apply the oil all over the body with light strokes, covering yourself in a thin layer. After you have coated the body, return to your scalp for a vigorous head massage to awaken your senses (most of our sense organs are in the head and face) and to clear out any fogginess caused by heat or stagnation. Next rub lightly up and down on the long bones, and in a circular motion around the joints. Remember to move clockwise around the belly, up and down the spine as best you can, and gently around the breasts and belly, under the arms, up and down the sides of your torso, and in a circular motion on the hips.

As you move down your thighs, take a moment to move around the knees (front and back), then the calves, ankles, toes, and tops of the feet, and then use whatever oil that remains on your hands to massage the soles of your feet. Make sure you don't use too much because you'll be rinsing off in the shower and you don't want it to be slippery.

Allow the oil to soak into the body for 15 or 20 minutes, if you can. I wear an old robe and perform other morning tasks while the oil sinks deep down through the layers of the tissues. Then, if you like, wipe off any oil that hasn't been absorbed—this is an optional step, but I like to do this, either with a towel or cloth used solely for this purpose. This ensures that only a very thin sheen of oil is left on my skin when I rinse off, so not too much goes down the drain.

Exercise...

In summer, we don't want to push ourselves to the max. Instead, think about working out just until you break a sweat and then slowing down a bit. Movement is always beneficial for flushing toxins out of our bodies, and in this season we also want to keep an eye toward moving heat out of the body.

In summer, yoga is an ideal way to work out. Traditional Hatha yoga is slow and mindful, flowing with the breath, paying attention to alignment, holding poses just long enough to adjust the body and feel the energy move from the tips of your toes to the crown of your head. Summer poses are designed to cool and calm the body and to reduce the urge to be competitive. Slow, mindful poses that open up the chest to allow cool air to easily flow in and out, and to expand the spine and align the body, are ideal—these poses include cat/cow, forward bends, camel, and fish. Twists are also great for squeezing Pitta (heat) out of the organs. Try windmills, side bends, and seated twists, twisting just as far as you are comfortable. Remember not to turn your chin past the shoulder. Align your gaze with the line of your navel. Don't force the pose. With each in-breath, lengthen your spine, resting on the out-breath. Stay in the twist for as long as it is comfortable, then slowly unwind and do the other side. Twisting and stretching moves Pitta out of the organs, intestines, and eyes. The movements should move excess heat from the body. Do not overheat or exercise to exhaustion. Avoid inversions, as we don't want heat to flow to the head. Avoid exercising in the heat of the day, from ten a.m. to two p.m.

No matter what exercise you do during Pitta season, be mindful of how you breathe! As Dr. John Douillard explains in his book *Mind, Body, Sport,* we breathe in two ways: diaphragmatic breathing and chest/clavicular breathing. Breathing from the diaphragm is optimal, especially when you exercise, since it facilitates a critical oxygenation process—but you can't reach that place in the lower ribs and lower lobes of the lungs when you breathe from your mouth! Always breathe through your nose—always.

Mouth breathing fills the chest and upper and middle lobes of the lungs, a shallow, emergency style of breathing that feels akin to the flight-or-fight response and has been linked to many illnesses.[12] Taking an emergency breath may be okay when you're being chased by a tiger, but it delivers insufficient oxygen for everyday living, let alone for exercise. Nose breathing, on the other hand, increases nitric oxide,[13] reduces stress and tension, activates our parasympathetic nervous system, and allows us to perform more work (exercise) with less effort.[14]

When you are working out, notice the moment when you feel you have to start breathing through your mouth—that is your "emergency breath" trigger. At that very moment, pull back a bit, slow down, lower the elevation on the treadmill, lessen the resistance on the bike or elliptical—slow down whatever it is you are doing. Continue breathing through your nose and once you have caught your breath and feel comfortable again, ramp up until you feel the urge to breathe through your mouth, then back down—over and over.

Over time you will notice that you can exercise hard while breathing more effectively through your nose, allowing the oxygen to flow completely through your body—not just the upper chest and lungs.

Essential Oils ....

Just by sniffing the oils you already have, or the ones at your local aromatherapy counter, you will notice immediately which scents relieve summer heat. I gravitate toward peppermint and lemon—probably recalling the "peppermint stick in the lemon" treat from my childhood—but other cooling oils include floral scents like jasmine, geranium, and rose; citrus scents like sweet orange, lime, and grapefruit; and, of course, the mints, peppermint and spearmint. Pure sandalwood oil, which is rare and hard to come by, is also excellent for Pitta season cooling.

Try placing a dot of oil on your forehead, at the base of your throat, and on your abdomen before work, going out, and meditation. You can also rub the soles of your feet and ankles with any of the above oils before bed.

Beyond scents, essential oils can be a powerful remedy or prevention for many of summer's ills. Take calendula, for example.[15] A homeopathic formula, calendula is the oil extracted from marigold flowers. Often mixed into creams for easy application, calendula oil has antifungal, anti-inflammatory, and antibacterial properties. It can be used for healing wounds, soothing eczema, and even relieving diaper rash, and it is a natural antiseptic. The cooling cream begins to heal the moment you put it on your skin, and I recommend it regularly to relieve itchy skin, hives, and bug bites, and in combination with aloe vera for sunburn.

Speaking of bug bites, using a natural insect repellant in summer is a must![16] I use the blends below for myself *and* my dogs (though check on flea and tick prevention with your veterinarian). Just be careful not to get any in your eyes or your pooch's.

ESSENTIAL OILS TO REPEL PESTS

MOSQUITOS: citronella, lemon, eucalyptus, peppermint, lemongrass, geranium, lavender (use 5 to 7 drops of each oil)

FLEAS: cedar wood, citronella, eucalyptus, tea tree, lemongrass, lavender, orange, pine

TICKS: rose geranium, juniper, rosewood, thyme, grapefruit, oregano

Pour 1/4 cup distilled water into a 4-ounce spray bottle, then add 1 ounce witch hazel and about 50 drops (total) of essential oils, based on the list above. You can also add about

1/2 ounce of a carrier oil to help rub the mix into your skin. If you find the blend is not strong enough, you can add a few more drops of essential oil. Stored in a glass or stainless-steel container in a cool, dark place, the pest repellant should last for up to a year or two.

In Ayurveda, the rose is known as a cooling flower, which makes it the perfect scent to use in summer.

Rose oil has been used medicinally for centuries.[17] It was revered in ancient Egypt and Iran and among Native Americans for its ability to heal many ailments, due to the high level of phenolic compounds it contains. Rose oil has been used to soothe sore throats, coughs, inflammation, and abdominal and chest pains. The oil is said to be an antidepressant, and can help to alleviate grief, stress, and tension. Rose oil can also heal skin wounds. Studies have also shown a reduction of blood pressure and increased feelings of calm and relaxation among those using rose oil.[18] You can store rose oil in a glass or stainless-steel container in a cool, dark place for up to a year.

Some Pitta/summer ailments, including headache and allergies, can be treated with rose hydrosol or rose oil spray. The spray will not only cool you down on a hot day, but it will also reduce skin irritation, remove redness, and help to balance your skin's natural pH.

DIY Rose Oil Hydrosol

To make your own spray, you just need a glass or stainless-steel spray bottle, some distilled water, and organic rose essential oil, a rose oil blend, or rose petals. Be sure to shake vigorously before using to mix the water and oil. Or you can get really serious[19] and purchase a professional hydrosol distiller.[20]

IF USING OIL, fill a spray bottle with room-temperature distilled water and add 10 to 15 drops of rose oil or rose oil blend. Seal and shake to mix.

IF USING ROSE PETALS, remove the petals from 7 to 10 roses and rinse under warm water to remove any debris. Place the petals in a small pot and add distilled water just to cover. Bring to a boil, then reduce the heat and simmer for about 20 minutes, until the petals are pale. If you need to, add more water to keep the petals covered. Remove from the heat and strain the rose water through cheesecloth into a bowl. Using a funnel, pour the rose water directly into the spray bottle.

Spritz the hydrosol onto your skin or hair. I love to carry a bottle with me all summer long to spray my face and neck anytime I need a quick cool down. I also like to spray my sheets and pillow before bed. You can also use this as a whole-body spray after a shower or bath. Store the spray at room temperature, or keep it in the refrigerator for an extra-cooling experience.

SUMMER SHIFTS TO FALL

Late summer is such a beautiful time of year when the heat begins to fade, the mornings have a chill to them, and the sun is shimmering white instead of a blazing golden yellow. The succulence of summer begins to dry out as we touch on the cusp of Vata season. Keep the body primed by ingesting healthy oils, and begin to eat warmer foods. Keep a cotton scarf or lightweight sweater with you, as the days and nights can be unpredictably cool. As we begin to wear more clothes, notice if you are feeling a bit more introspective; perhaps you have the urge to call it a night earlier and you crave a cup of golden milk (see page 152) before bed. Allow yourself to give in to these urges even if the temperature is still warm outside. It's the body's natural reaction to Pitta time coming to an end and Vata time unfolding. Pay attention to those natural urges as you are now more in tune with the seasons. Listen to your body and mind and you may notice the change of season brings on a shift in energy. Exercise can become a bit more vigorous. Meditation has more intention. The body craves more cooked food and less raw.

Even before the date on the calendar says it's autumn, you can begin to squirrel away your nuts and seeds and ready yourself for the harvest to come.

CONCLUSION

The Years Cycle On

Ayurveda is the science of life—and I consider it a *living* science of life. The knowledge of Ayurveda is an ancient stream that flows with fresh water that we can drink from as needed. Hopefully you will take a dip in the stream, or even immerse yourself totally, and allow yourself to flow with the healing waters. By now you've embraced a year of self-care rituals aimed at bringing you into balance with each season, and I hope you can take a moment to notice all that has changed during the previous months, and what you will look forward to in the months and years ahead.

You now know which doshas have accumulated at the end of the season, and which daily routines to take on in order to reduce the buildup, create a clean slate, and usher you into the new season. You can use food to heal and bolster your immunity, as well as to prevent damage from toxins getting into your body. With regular meditation you will begin to see the world, and your place in it, differently. Barriers will come down, and you will discover strength in vulnerability and learn to love yourself exactly as you are. As you practice breathing, you will notice incredible reduction in your stress level, improved digestion, increased stamina, and the deep relaxation that comes from activating the parasympathetic nervous system. Be aware of your gut and skin microbiome and the essential roles they play in your good health. And remember to stay in touch with your energy body. Check in with your chakras to see what needs care and tuning, and use the practices here accordingly. With all these habits in place, sleep should come naturally, and you will feel rested and restored each morning.

You will be aware now of when you have too much heat, too much cold, or too much dampness, and—more important—you will know what to do about it! If you wake up feeling lethargic and unrested, you will remember to think about what happened the day before: What and when did you eat? Where did you go? Did you take time for yourself? Now you will be able to clearly discern where you may have gone astray, and you know how to fix it.

And if you don't remember, don't worry! Think of *Seasonal Self-Care Rituals* as your perennial guide to well-being and seasonal harmony. The recommendations and ideas contained here are based on wisdom that has not changed in thousands of years—our task is to understand, adjust, and fine-tune these routines to accommodate our needs. You can and should refer back to these chapters often, trying on new rituals, adopting new practices, and employing new remedies at the change of each season. Don't give up—you are always welcome to come back and pick up where you left off.

I suggest making copies of the seasonal grocery lists and keeping those handy. When you think of a recipe you want to make, look at the foods for the season and see what works for you. Plan some menus. Stock the pantry each season with rice, quinoa, millet, canned and dried beans, nut butters, nuts and seeds, and ghee and other oils—according to your dosha. Buy an Indian spice tray so you can store your spice churnas and other spices you use daily. Every kitchen in India has one, and they're easy to find online. With all your spices in one place, cooking is a breeze. You can store leftover spices in airtight containers and refill the spice tray as needed.

Do whatever you need to do to make your daily rituals easy. For example, I have a low bench in my bathroom on which I store my electric kettle and all my Ayurvedic herbs, oils, and tinctures. If it wasn't handy first thing in the morning, I might be tempted to skip over it. Look around your home and think about how you can create a space for your self-care ritual bench or cabinet.

You can do the same for your meditation space. Find an area tucked away from the rest of the world. We know facing east is best in the morning, but being in a quiet, settled area is most important. For me that's often the guest bedroom, with maybe a dog or two snoring on the bed, but I know people who meditate in their closet! The key is to find what works for you and create sacred space for yourself by literally setting up a place for these acts of self-care.

Whatever it is, find what works for you. If you don't, you won't do it—it's that simple! Take your time. Committing to your seasonal self-care rituals can lead you to a rich new world with an open mind. I hope you will use this book as a springboard to well-being and self-fulfillment. Once we clear the path of toxins and other obstacles that may have been in our way, our spirit can soar. With balanced doshas, you can move beyond the day-to-day planning and into a reality filled with unlimited potential.

Maybe you have been inspired to deepen your knowledge of Ayurveda—it is so rich, layered, and complex that it can take a lifetime of study and practice to master all the skills. But what you have learned here will set you up for success and allow you to reap the benefits right away. To continue your studies of Ayurveda, please see the resources guide that begins on page 175.

It is exciting to know that you can heal yourself and that *you* are in charge of your own well-being. Ayurveda will be here for you, just as it has been for more than five thousand years. These ideas of living in harmony with the natural world are not going anywhere. Use your imagination to invent new and creative ways to balance your doshas—the Universe is always providing us with inspiration and potentiality. As you age, take these concepts with you and adjust them as needed.

I want you to see the beauty in every season of your life. The boundless energy and enthusiasm of youth may be tinged with uncertainty and fear. But that will bloom into a stage of life with more certainty, fortitude, and drive. As you grow in your career, family life, relationships, watch for each dosha so you will know where you stand—and also to better understand those around you. Lean into the later years when creativity unfolds, when you know yourself even better and you can fly free from the "rules" (if you ever followed them to begin with!).

I am so happy you found this book, and I am filled with joy knowing that you have this power for change at your fingertips. Live your life to the fullest and enjoy all it has to offer you. Eat, breathe, move, meditate, and sleep well. Happiness is within you.

APPENDIX A

Seasonal Grocery Lists

These grocery lists have been adapted from *The 3-Season Diet* by John Douillard (Three Rivers Press, 2000) and *The Ayurvedic Cookbook* by Amadea Morningstar (Lotus Press, 1992).

As always, please try to buy or grow organic! Local is good, but even at the farmers' market be sure to ask your vendors whether their crops were sprayed with nonorganic pesticides like glyphosate (aka Roundup). If they were, move on, or remember to wash all of your produce *really* well.

Make copies of these seasonal grocery lists and keep them with you when you go shopping. If you live in an area where it is difficult to find fresh produce, do your best with canned and frozen foods. Just check the ingredients for added sugar, salt, or preservatives, and try to steer clear of those. Other items like beans, lentils, rice, grains, seeds, and spices can easily be found online. Many areas do not have an Indian store nearby, but some of these items can be found in Middle Eastern, Asian, or Korean markets as well as online. Explore! You will be amazed at some of the hidden gems in your neighborhood. Maybe you can even plant a garden for greens, beans, and other produce.

VATA SEASON GROCERY LIST

Fruits ....

- Apples (cooked)
- Apricots (if dried, soak before using)
- Avocados
- Bananas
- Cantaloupe
- Dates
- Figs
- Grapefruit
- Grapes
- Lemons
- Limes
- Oranges
- Papaya
- Prunes
- Tangerines

Vegetables ....

- Beets
- Brussels sprouts
- Carrots
- Chiles
- Corn
- Eggplant
- Garlic
- Green beans
- Leeks
- Onions
- Okra
- Parsley
- Potatoes
- Pumpkin
- Root vegetables
- Seaweed (cook before consuming)
- Spinach (cooked)
- Sweet potatoes
- Winter squash

Grains ....

- Amaranth
- Barley
- Buckwheat
- Corn
- Millet
- Oats
- Rice, white or wild
- Rye
- Seitan
- Wheat

Legumes ....

- Miso paste
- Mung beans
- Tempeh
- Tofu
- Urad dal

Nuts and Seeds ....

- Almonds
- Brazil nuts
- Cashews
- Hazelnuts
- Macadamia nuts
- Peanuts
- Pecans
- Pine nuts
- Pistachios
- Walnuts
- Sunflower seeds

Dairy..

- Butter
- Cottage cheese
- Cow's milk (not cold)
- Feta cheese
- Ghee
- Goat's milk (not cold)
- Soft cheeses
- Sour cream

Animal Proteins.......................................

- Beef
- Chicken
- Crab
- Duck
- Eggs
- Freshwater fish
- Pork
- Oysters
- Shrimp
- Turkey
- Venison

Oils ....

- Almond
- Avocado
- Canola
- Coconut
- Flaxseed
- Ghee
- Mustard
- Olive
- Sesame
- Safflower
- Sunflower

Sweeteners...

- Honey
- Jaggery
- Molasses
- Rice syrup
- Sucanat

KAPHA SEASON GROCERY LIST

Fruits ....

- Apples
- Apricots
- Apricots, dried
- Blueberries
- Cherries
- Cranberries
- Dried fruit
- Lemons
- Limes
- Peaches
- Pears
- Pomegranates
- Prunes
- Raisins
- Raspberries
- Strawberries

Vegetables ....

- Artichokes
- Asparagus
- Bell peppers
- Beets and beet greens
- Bitter gourd (aka karela)
- Broccoli
- Brussels sprouts
- Cabbage
- Carrots
- Cauliflower (all colors)
- Celery
- Chard
- Chiles
- Collard greens
- Corn
- Dandelion greens
- Endive
- Garlic
- Green beans
- Kale
- Leeks
- Lettuce
- Mushrooms
- Mustard greens
- Onions
- Peas
- Potatoes (purple, white, or russet)
- Radishes
- Spinach
- Turnips

Grains/Seeds......................................

- Amaranth
- Barley
- Buckwheat
- Corn
- Millet
- Oats (dry, not cooked)
- Popcorn (with Spring Spice Churna; page 76 or 154)
- Pumpkin seeds, unsalted
- Quinoa
- Rice, basmati
- Rice cakes
- Rye
- Seitan
- Sunflower seeds, unsalted

Legumes ....

- Adzuki beans
- Black beans
- Black-eyed peas
- Chickpeas (aka garbanzo beans)
- Kidney beans
- Lima beans
- Lentils
- Miso paste
- Mung beans
- Navy beans
- Pinto beans
- Tempeh
- Toor dal
- White beans

Animal Proteins......................................

- Eggs
- Fish, freshwater
- Poultry (white meat)
- Rabbit
- Shrimp
- Venison

Dairy...

(Only if you do not have a Kapha imbalance. Avoid dairy completely if
Kapha is very high.)

- Cottage cheese
- Goat's milk

- Yogurt, plain, full-fat

Oils ....

- Flaxseed
- Ghee
- Mustard

- Safflower
- Sunflower

Spices ....

- All spices

Sweeteners...

- Honey
- Jaggery

- Maple syrup, pure
- Molasses

PITTA SEASON GROCERY LIST

Fruits ....

(Look for sweet, ripe, juicy fruits, melons, and berries.)

- Apples (sweet, not sour)
- Avocados
- Berries
- Cherries
- Coconut
- Cranberries
- Grapes
- Limes
- Mangoes
- Melons
- Pears
- Pineapples
- Plums
- Pomegranates
- Prunes

Vegetables ....

(Leafy greens continue the detoxification process begun in spring. Try not to eat raw.)

- Artichokes
- Arugula
- Asparagus
- Beet greens
- Bok choy
- Broccoli
- Brussels sprouts
- Cabbage
- Cauliflower (all colors)
- Celery
- Chard
- Collard greens
- Cucumbers
- Dandelion greens
- Endive
- Green beans
- Kale
- Lettuce
- Microgreens
- Mizuna
- Okra
- Potatoes
- Radicchio
- Watercress
- Zucchini

Grains ....

- Barley
- Farro
- Quinoa
- Rice (white basmati)
- Wheat

Legumes ....

- Adzuki beans
- Black beans
- Chickpeas (aka garbanzo beans)
- Mung beans
- Split peas

Oils ....

- Coconut oil (high heat)
- Flaxseed (cold)
- Ghee (in moderation)
- Hemp seed (cold)
- Olive oil (low to medium heat)
- Sunflower (medium heat)
- Udo's Oil (omega 3-6-9 blend, cold)

Herbs and Spices.....................................

- Basil
- Cardamom
- Cilantro
- Cinnamon
- Coriander
- Dill
- Fennel
- Lime
- Mint
- Parsley

Animal Proteins......................................

- Fish (freshwater)
- Poultry (white meat)
- Shrimp

Dairy...
(Stick to nondairy versions if you can and look for vegan options.)

- Feta cheese (in moderation)
- Goat cheese (in moderation)
- Hemp milk
- Oat milk
- Coconut milk
- Coconut milk ice cream

Sweeteners..

- Coconut palm sugar
- Jaggery
- Maple syrup, pure
- Monk fruit
- Sucanat
- Yacon syrup

APPENDIX B

Seasonal Recipes

VATA SEASON

Food is a huge part of our seasonal traditions and rituals, and we can often run into trouble during the winter season when there are so many holidays and gatherings. Following Ayurvedic guidelines for the season doesn't mean that you can't enjoy meals with family and friends. These recipes offer the perfect remedy for the cold, dry season by substituting winter-friendly spices, vegetables, oils, and more to help you stay balanced.

VATA SEASON SPICE MIX

1 tablespoon coriander seeds
1 tablespoon cumin seeds
2 tablespoons fennel seeds
2 tablespoons ginger powder
1 tablespoon turmeric powder
1 tablespoon dried basil
1 teaspoon sea salt
1/2 teaspoon hing (asafœtida)

Combine all the spices in a spice grinder or clean coffee grinder
and grind. Spoon the ground spice mix into a clean glass jar or
stainless-steel container with a lid. Make sure there is a tight seal
on the container. The spices contain essential oils that we want
to keep stable. Best used within 1 year to assure the freshness of
the healing essential oils in the spices. Store in a cool, dark place.
You can fill a small jar to carry with you when you eat out.

NO-EGG EGG NOG

This very grounding recipe is actually a great energy booster throughout the season, as both dates and cashews are Vata-pacifying. Pitta and Kapha can take this drink in moderation.

SERVES 2

2 cups cashew milk, macadamia nut milk, or almond milk (plain or unsweetened vanilla)

1/2 cup full-fat canned coconut milk

1/3 cup raw cashews, soaked overnight or for at least 30 minutes (optional)

4 to 6 Medjool dates, pitted

1/2 teaspoon pure vanilla extract

1/2 teaspoon pure almond extract

1/2 teaspoon freshly grated nutmeg, plus more for serving if desired

Pinch of ground cinnamon, plus more for serving if desired

Pinch of ground cloves

Pinch of sea salt

Combine all the ingredients in a high-speed blender and blend until smooth and creamy. Serve immediately, with a pinch of nutmeg or cinnamon on top.

VEGAN SUPERFOOD PUMPKIN CASHEW CHIA PUDDING

This "creamy" concoction will leave you wondering where the dairy is. The benefits of being dairy-free create a treat that is easier to digest, lighter, and warmer than heavy milk, cream, or eggs. The pumpkin is nutrient-dense with a lot of fiber, making it a great food for the colder season. The nuts are also warming, with a huge amount of protein. And chia seeds create moisture as well as being a nutritional superfood. This all adds up to a perfect treat to indulge in during the winter season.

SERVES 8

1/4 cup chia seeds, soaked and drained

1/2 cup raw unsalted cashews, soaked for at least 1 hour

2 cups organic pure pumpkin puree (canned or see Note to make your own)

1 teaspoon pure vanilla extract

2 Medjool dates, pitted

2 teaspoons pure maple syrup

1 teaspoon mixed ground spices (cardamom, cinnamon, cloves, ginger, nutmeg)

Freshly grated nutmeg, for garnish

In a high-speed blender, combine the chia seeds, cashews, pumpkin, vanilla, dates, maple syrup, and spices and blend until smooth and creamy. Pour into a large bowl or individual serving cups. Garnish with freshly grated nutmeg and serve.

NOTE: *Homemade Pumpkin Puree*—Preheat the oven to 350°F. Cut a medium pumpkin in half and remove the seeds and stringy pulp. Coat the flesh with coconut oil and place both halves facedown on a baking sheet. Roast for 45 minutes, until the flesh is tender and easily pierced with a fork. Remove from the oven and let cool, then scoop out the flesh and mash until smooth. Makes about 4 cups pumpkin puree.

VEGAN CREAMED
SPINACH AND CAULIFLOWER

Blending is a delightful way to enjoy vegetables this time of year. The warm, creamy sensation reminds me of hearty winter foods. You can substitute root vegetables like sweet potatoes and beets for the cauliflower, and other greens like chard or kale that you may have on hand in place of the spinach.

SERVES 4 TO 6
2 cups chopped cauliflower (about one-half of a small head)
2/3 cup unsweetened nondairy milk
2 tablespoons olive oil or avocado oil
1 medium onion, finely chopped
3 medium garlic cloves, minced
1/2 teaspoon freshly grated nutmeg
1 pound spinach, washed well and coarsely chopped
Salt and freshly ground black pepper

In a 4-quart soup pot, combine the cauliflower and milk and bring to a simmer over medium heat, then reduce the heat to the lowest setting, cover, and cook until the cauliflower is completely tender, about 10 minutes. Using an immersion blender, puree the cauliflower until smooth (or carefully transfer the contents of the pot to a countertop blender and puree). Set aside.

In a large saucepan, heat the oil over medium heat. Add the onion and cook, stirring frequently, until softened but not browned, about 4 minutes. Add the garlic and cook, stirring continuously, until fragrant, about 30 seconds. Add the nutmeg and stir. Add the spinach one handful at a time, stirring and folding until each handful of spinach is wilted before adding the next.

Add the cauliflower puree to the pan and stir to combine. Bring to a simmer and cook, stirring occasionally, until the spinach is completely tender and the mixture is creamy. Taste, season with salt and pepper, and serve.

ORANGE WALNUT DATE DESSERT

I first enjoyed this yummy treat while on a cooking retreat with Amadea Morningstar. She tossed some dates into a pan with ghee and we stuffed them with a walnuts or almonds. It was so delicious I took it on as my own over the years and added the orange juice for Vata season—but credit is due where credit is due! It's the perfect way to end a meal, or enjoy it with a warm cup of tea.

SERVES 4

1 to 2 tablespoons ghee (clarified butter), or walnut oil or coconut oil (for a vegan version), plus more as needed

1/3 cup orange juice, plus more as needed

12 to 16 Medjool dates, pitted

12 to 16 walnuts (halves or whole pieces)

Unsweetened shredded coconut, for coating (optional)

In a large skillet, melt the ghee over medium heat. Add the orange juice and stir together.

Add the dates and stir to coat them well. Cook until fully heated through, 3 to 4 minutes, then transfer the dates to a plate and let cool. (If the dates stick to the pan, you can add more ghee and OJ as needed.)

When the dates are cool enough to touch, stuff each with a walnut, then close the date around it.

If desired, place some shredded coconut in a bowl and roll the stuffed dates in the coconut to coat lightly. Arrange the dates on a plate and serve.

WINTER VEGETABLE KITCHARI

This Ayurvedic staple is the perfect winter meal. It was the
first Ayurvedic recipe I learned, and after eating just one
bite, I knew I had found my calling. The blend of split yellow mung beans, basmati rice, ghee, spices, and vegetables
is the most satisfying meal, as all your needs are met here
in one dish! Select just one or two veggies for each pot
you make, and try to make it fresh every day. Kitchari is a
complete protein, texturally satisfying, and filled with heating
spices and ghee for absorbing all the nutrients.

SERVES 4

1/2 cup dried split yellow mung beans (moong dal)
1/2 cup uncooked white basmati rice
1 to 2 cups vegetables of your choice (squash, green beans,
     beets, mustard greens, okra, daikon radish, carrots, peas,
     sweet potatoes)

1 (1-inch) piece fresh ginger, peeled and grated or minced
1 teaspoon sea salt (see Notes)
1/2 teaspoon freshly ground black pepper
1 teaspoon ghee, for serving (optional)
Bragg Liquid Aminos, for serving (optional)
1 tablespoon fresh cilantro or parsley, chopped,
     for garnish (optional)

FOR THE VAGAR (OIL-SPICE MIX)

2 tablespoons ghee
1 teaspoon black mustard seeds

1 teaspoon ground turmeric

1/2 teaspoon cumin seeds

1/2 teaspoon ground coriander

1/2 teaspoon ajwain (carom seeds; available at any Indian grocery store

Pinch of hing (asafœtida)

Rinse the beans and rice together until the water runs clear, and let them sit in the water while you prepare the vegetables and vagar.

Meanwhile, prep the vegetables: Wash well and chop them into bite-size pieces.

Make the oil/spice mix (vagar): Turn on your exhaust fan over the stove, as the scent of the spices will be strong. In an 8-quart soup pot, melt the ghee over medium-high heat. Add the mustard seeds. When they pop, add the turmeric, cumin, coriander, ajwain, and hing and cook until aromatic, about 1 minute. Spices burn quickly, so make sure the vagar doesn't begin to smoke! If it does, just lower the heat.

Stir in the ginger. Drain the beans and rice. Add them to the pot and stir to coat with the vagar, then cook, stirring occasionally, for 45 seconds to 1 minute. Add 4 to 6 cups water (see Notes) and stir. Stir in the vegetables. Cover and bring to a boil, then reduce the heat to maintain a simmer and cook until all the water has been absorbed, about 15 minutes, or until the kitchari is the consistency you prefer. (You can place the lid askew to let out steam, as this lets out extra Vata.) Toward the end of the cooking time, season with the salt and pepper. Remove from the heat.

Place your portion in a bowl. If desired, top with the ghee as well as a splash of liquid aminos and garnish with the cilantro or parsley. Store leftovers in an airtight container in the refrigerator for no more than 24 hours. To reheat, add some water to the uneaten portions in the pot and cook over medium heat until hot. (Never freeze or reheat in the microwave.)

NOTES: *It's important to use sea salt for the extra moisture provided. Do not use Himalayan salt in this recipe; it is too "dry" for Vata season.*

Use less water for a stewlike consistency or more water for a soupier consistency.

GOLDEN MILK FOR
SLEEP AND GOOD DIGESTION

This elixir has been used for centuries to deeply nourish the tissues and replenish the bodily constituents. It's excellent for ensuring a good night's rest and a healthy bowel movement in the morning. It is balancing for all three doshas (Kapha benefits most using the vegan version). There are many recipes for golden milk out there, but I like this very simple version. You can use this any time you have trouble sleeping, no matter the season.

SERVES 1

1 cup milk of your choice
1 teaspoon ghee
1/2 teaspoon ground turmeric
Pinch of ground cinnamon
Pinch of ground nutmeg
Pinch of freshly ground black pepper
Pinch of ground ginger
1 teaspoon jaggery (optional)

In a small saucepan, heat the milk over medium heat until just boiling, then reduce the heat to maintain a simmer. Add the ghee, turmeric, cinnamon, nutmeg, pepper, ginger, and jaggery (if using), and whisk to combine. Remove from the heat.

Pour the golden milk into your favorite mug and sip while engaging in restful activities.

RECIPES FOR KAPHA SEASON

SPRING SPICE CHURNA

1 tablespoon ground ginger
1 tablespoon freshly ground black pepper
1 tablespoon ground coriander
1 tablespoon ground turmeric
1 teaspoon Himalayan salt
1 tablespoon ground cinnamon
Pinch of cayenne pepper

Mix the spices together in a spice grinder or coffee grinder.
Pour into a glass or stainless steel container with a tight lid.
Store in a cool, dark place for up to 1 year. You can use this
at home for cooking and take it with you when you eat out.
It will not only make your food taste more delicious, but it
will help to balance Kapha dosha in the spring or any time
Kapha needs reducing.

SPRING TEA

Spring tea can be any blend of herbs that contain pungent, bitter and astringent qualities will help to reduce congestion, stuffiness and lethargy we can feel in springtime. These teas will also help to shed the accumulated Kapha we put on in winter. Choose from the following herbs or spices, ready-made blends, or make your own!

Ginger	Cayenne pepper
Peppermint	Cumin
Tulsi	Fennel
Clove	Black pepper
Cinnamon	Licorice
Cardamom	Fenugreek
Turmeric	

Try the "other" CCF (cumin, coriander, fennel) tea for spring:

2 pods cardamom
1/2 teaspoon coriander seeds
1/2 teaspoon fennel seeds

Steep the seeds in 3 cups just-boiled water. Strain into a mug and sip throughout the day. You can add more hot water as needed. I use the same seeds for 3 or 4 cups of tea. *Optional:* If you have spring allergies, add 1/2 teaspoon stinging nettles to the mix, or drink stinging nettle tea on its own during the allergy season.

SPRING DETOX SOUP

This is my favorite soup in spring—I have been known to eat a bowl for breakfast, lunch, and dinner! The greens help to remove toxins from the body, while the spices will heat up and melt accumulated gunk left over from the winter. The veggies are filled with nutrients. This is a complete meal.

SERVES 4

2 carrots, sliced and diced
2 celery stalks, chopped
2 or 3 garlic cloves, smashed and finely chopped
4 bok choy leaves, chopped
1/2 cup daikon radish, sliced and diced
2 dried red chiles (optional)
2 or 3 curry leaves or bay leaves (optional)
1 tablespoon chopped fresh ginger
Freshly ground black pepper
1 small bunch dandelion greens, chopped
1 cup coconut milk (optional, benefits Pitta)
Juice of 1 large lime
2 tablespoons tamari
Himalayan salt (optional; see Note)
Ghee (optional, benefits Vata and Pitta)

Bring 8 cups water (or 7 cups, if you'll be adding coconut milk later) to a boil in a large soup pot. Add the carrots, celery, garlic, bok choy, daikon, dried chiles (if using), and curry leaves (if using). Add the ginger and season with pepper. Reduce the heat to low, cover, and simmer for 10 to 15 minutes, until the vegetables are lightly cooked.

Stir in the dandelion greens and the coconut milk (if using). Remove from the heat and add the lime juice and tamari. Taste and season with salt, if desired.

Pour into bowls and serve hot. For Vata and Pitta, add 1 teaspoon ghee per bowl before serving.

NOTE: It is important to use Himalayan salt as it is a mountain salt and dry, as opposed to sea salt, which is moist.

KAPHA SEASON KITCHARI

This recipe gives the option to use quinoa instead of kitchari's more traditional rice base. Quinoa is a light seed, full of protein and nutrients, and is very easy to digest—perfect for spring. You can also use this recipe for a cleanse as a mono diet. Just eat this for three days for breakfast, lunch, and dinner!

SERVES 4

1/2 cup dried split yellow mung beans (moong dal)
1/2 cup uncooked white basmati rice or quinoa
1 small yellow onion, chopped
1 (2-inch) piece fresh ginger, peeled and grated or minced

1 or 2 garlic cloves, chopped

1/2 teaspoon Himalayan salt (see Notes, page 160) or lemon
   salt, if you can find it

1 teaspoon freshly ground black pepper

2 carrots, chopped

2 celery stalks, chopped

1 cup chopped mixed vegetables and/or leafy greens (two or
   three types; see Notes, page 160)

1 teaspoon Bragg Liquid Aminos (optional)

Small handful of fresh cilantro, chopped, for garnish (optional)

FOR THE VAGAR (OIL-SPICE MIX)

1 teaspoon ghee

1 teaspoon black mustard seeds

1 teaspoon ground turmeric

1/2 teaspoon cumin seeds

1/2 teaspoon ground coriander

1/2 teaspoon ajwain (carom seeds)

1/2 teaspoon ground cinnamon

1/2 teaspoon ground cloves, or 2 or 3 whole cloves

Pinch of hing (asafœtida)

Rinse the beans and rice (or quinoa) together until the water
runs relatively clear. This mix can soak while you prepare the
rest of the recipe.

Make the oil/spice mix (vagar): Turn on your exhaust
fan over the stove, as the scent of the spices will be strong.
In an 4- or 6-quart soup pot, melt the ghee over medium-
high heat. Add the mustard seeds. When they pop, add the
turmeric, cumin, coriander, ajwain, cinnamon, cloves, and hing

and cook until aromatic, about 1 minute. Spices burn quickly, so make sure the vagar doesn't begin to smoke!

Stir in the onion, ginger, and garlic. Drain the rice (or quinoa) and beans. Add them to the pot and stir to coat with the vagar, then cook, stirring occasionally, for 45 seconds to 1 minute. Add 4 to 6 cups water and stir (see Notes below). Stir in the vegetables. Cover and bring to a boil over medium-high heat, then reduce the heat to maintain a simmer and cook until all the water has been absorbed, about 15 minutes, or until the kitchari is the consistency you prefer. Toward the end of the cooking time, season with the salt and pepper. Add the carrots, celery, and mixed vegetables and/or greens and stir until wilted, then remove from the heat.

Place your portion in a bowl. If desired, add the liquid aminos and garnish with the cilantro. Store leftovers in the refrigerator for no more than 24 hours. To reheat, add some water to the uneaten portions in the pot and heat over medium heat until hot. (Never freeze or reheat in the microwave.)

NOTES: *Ideal vegetable choices for this dish include burdock root, asparagus, cauliflower, broccoli, white potato, daikon radish, green beans, spinach, kale, mustard greens, and chard.*

Use less water for a stewlike consistency or more water for a soupier consistency.

It is important to use Himalayan salt in this recipe; sea salt will add more water to already watery Kapha, which is undesired.

RAMPED-UP ROASTED RAMPS

One of the gifts of spring I wait for every year is ramps. These alliums are kind of like a scallion, kind of like a leek, and kind of like a spring onion—but they're actually none of those things! Ramps have a tiny white bulb on the end of long, broad, flat leaves. Their garlicky flavor instantly adds another layer to whatever you are cooking. They grow just on the cusp of winter and spring, making them one of the first wild harbingers of the season. Ramps are loaded with vitamin C and go well with just about everything savory on the menu. I love them roasted, combined with spring vegetables or gluten-free pasta, or just on their own out of the pan!

SERVES 2 AS MAIN OR 4 AS A SIDE

1 cup Brussels sprouts
2 white potatoes, scrubbed and very thinly sliced
Avocado oil
Pinch of ground cumin
Pinch of ground ginger
Maldon sea salt or other flaky salt
10 to 15 ramps
1 endive

Preheat the oven to 450°F.

Trim the Brussels sprouts, remove and discard their outer leaves, and cut them in half (or quarter them, if large). Spread the sprouts and the potatoes in a single layer over the bottom of a baking pan. Cover with a thin layer of avocado oil and sprinkle with the cumin, ginger, and some flaky salt. Use your hands or a spoon to mix the veggies with the oil and spices to coat (these spices help make the potatoes more digestible). Roast for 30 to 35 minutes, turning them once halfway through.

Meanwhile, place the ramps and endive in a second baking pan. Cover with a thin layer of avocado oil and sprinkle with flaky salt. When the potatoes and sprouts have been in the oven for 20 to 25 minutes, place the pan with the ramps in the oven as well. Roast for 10 to 15 minutes, until the leaves of the ramps and endive are slightly charred.

Remove both pans from the oven. Transfer all the vegetables to a serving dish, toss to combine, and serve warm.

CELERY BEET-DOWN TOXINS JUICE

I only use my juicer in late spring and summer when agni is low—the digestive fires are set on a slow burn so that we can stay cooler without depleting our energy. During this time of year, I naturally feel less hungry, so juice often does the trick as a meal. In the fall and winter when I feel hungrier and agni is high, I prefer to eat food that has all of its fiber intact. Juicing removes fiber and produces just the liquid of the fruit or vegetable. Without the fiber, the juice has an immediate impact on the system and is easily absorbed into the bloodstream, providing a big energy boost. Juicing is also great for people who are ill or have compromised immune systems, as the body doesn't need to work so hard to get the nutrients. Use this juice as a meal replacement, or drink it on an empty stomach about 1 hour before a light meal.

SERVES 2

1 bunch celery (6 to 8 stalks)
1 small beet
1 (1-inch) piece fresh ginger
1/2 lime
1/2 cup fresh cilantro

Wash all the ingredients well. (No need to peel the beet, ginger, or lime—just give them a good scrub.) Pass all the ingredients through a juicer into a pitcher and stir, if needed. Drink immediately, or pour into an airtight container, refrigerate, and consume within the next few hours.

RECIPES FOR PITTA SEASON

SUMMER SPICE CHURNA

Handful of crushed fresh or dried mint leaves
2 tablespoons coriander seeds
2 tablespoons cumin seeds
2 tablespoons fennel seeds
1 tablespoon green cardamom seeds
1 tablespoon ground turmeric
1 teaspoon ground cinnamon
1 teaspoon ground ginger
1 teaspoon coconut palm sugar, Sucanat, or jaggery
1/2 teaspoon sea salt

Combine all the ingredients in a spice grinder or blender and grind to a powder. Transfer to a glass jar or other airtight container. Store in a cool, dark place for up to 1 year. Add to any savory foods. Fill a small container to take with you when you eat out.

FLORAL SUMMER SALT BLEND

In a blender, combine equal amounts of mineral salt, dried organic rose petals, and dried hibiscus flowers and pulse until the rose petals and hibiscus are powdered. The resulting salt will be a deep shade of pink. Store in a saltshaker and use as needed in place of table salt, at home and when you eat out.

MINTY LIME BASIL FENNEL JUICE

Nearly all the tastes to balance summer are in this drink. The lime skin will give the juice a refreshing hint of bitterness, the apples are sweet, the celery is a bit salty, and the basil and fennel add fuel and can be both stimulating and cooling.

SERVES 2
4 Pink Lady or Fuji apples
1 lime
1 small handful of basil (about 10 leaves)
1/2 small fennel bulb
2 celery stalks

Wash all the ingredients well. (No need to peel the apples or lime—just give them a good scrub and core the apple to remove the seeds.) Pass all the ingredients through a juicer into a pitcher and stir, if needed. Drink immediately, or pour into an airtight container, refrigerate, and drink within 12 hours for maximum health benefits.

VERY BERRY SMOOTHIE

Traditionally, Ayurveda stays away from very cold food, as it will put out our digestive fires, hindering our ability to fully digest our food. How we work this out with the ever-popular smoothie is to stay away from frozen ingredients and use warm liquids. If you do use frozen berries in this recipe, soak them first in hot water. Use any combination of berries you have on hand for this smoothie—the types listed are just suggestions. Just be sure to use 2 cups berries total.

SERVES 2

1/2 cup blackberries
1/2 cup raspberries
1/2 cup blueberries
1/2 cup strawberries
1 to 2 teaspoons fresh mint leaves, or
    1/4 teaspoon pure mint extract
1/4 teaspoon ground cardamom, or 1 green cardamom pod
1 tablespoon unsweetened shredded coconut
1 teaspoon hemp or chia seeds
3/4 cup nondairy yogurt or nondairy milk (such as coconut, almond, or macadamia)
Optional add-ins (great for Pitta and Vata, not so much needed for Kapha): 1 teaspoon Udo's Oil or coconut oil, 1 scoop hemp powder or protein powder

Combine all the ingredients (including any optional add-ins) in a blender and blend for about 30 seconds, or until smooth. Add warm or room-temperature water, as needed, until you like the consistency. Enjoy right away!

NOTE: *Leave out the water and pour the extra-thick smoothie into a bowl to enjoy with a spoon.*

SUSAN'S SUMMER SMOOTHIE

While Ayurveda does not approve of frozen food, frozen organic fruits and vegetables can sometimes be more nutrient dense than those that have been trucked across the country and stored in a warehouse for days before they make their way out to the produce section. If you can't find organic local produce, I think using frozen organic—which is flash frozen very close to where it was harvested—is a fine choice.

SERVES 1

1 cup fresh berries (if frozen, thaw in hot water for a few minutes)
1 tablespoon Udo's Oil, coconut oil, or flax seed oil
1 tablespoon chia seeds
1/4 cup full-fat canned coconut milk
1 cup almond milk, warmed

Combine all the ingredients in a blender and whir it up for 30 seconds or so. Add warm or room-temperature water, as needed, until you like the consistency. Serve and enjoy!

MINTY CUCUMBER RAITA

Raita is traditionally used as a condiment to cool down hot, spicy Indian food. But you can enjoy it as a dish all on its own, serve it over a bowl of rice, or even use it as a dressing on a salad.

SERVES 4

2 to 3 small cucumbers (pickling cukes have more flavor)
1 cup dairy or nondairy, unsweetened, full-fat yogurt
1/4 teaspoon sea salt
1/4 teaspoon freshly ground black or white pepper
1/4 teaspoon ground cumin
Fresh mint leaves, for garnish

Using the large holes of a box grater, grate the cucumbers into a medium bowl. Add the yogurt, salt, pepper, and cumin and stir well to combine. If desired, transfer the raita to a blender and blend to the desired consistency (this will result in a smoother raita), then return the raita to a bowl. Garnish with mint leaves and serve.

CUCUMBER AVOCADO PINEAPPLE SALAD

This combination of fruits and veggies might seem a bit odd, but I promise you will love it! Cool, smooth, and creamy with a lime sparkle, it is the perfect summer salad. The combination of spices helps to make this dish easily digestible. And with the optional addition of cannellini beans, this becomes a protein-rich meal!

SERVES 4

3 cucumbers, chopped into bite-size pieces

1 to 2 cups chopped pineapple

1 cup cooked or canned cannellini beans, drained (optional)

1/2 cup mixed fresh cilantro and parsley, finely chopped

2 scallions or small handful of fresh chives, chopped, or 1/4 cup
   diced red onion

Zest and juice of 1 lime

1 tablespoon extra-virgin olive oil or avocado oil, plus more as
   needed

Pinch of ground cumin

Sea salt and freshly ground black pepper

2 cups arugula

1/2 ripe avocado, cubed

In a medium bowl, combine the cucumbers, pineapple, beans (if using), cilantro-parsley mixture, scallions, lime zest, half of the lime juice, the olive oil, and the cumin. Season with salt and pepper and toss to combine.

In a serving bowl, toss the arugula with a bit of olive oil and the remaining lime juice. Spoon the cucumber-pineapple mix on top, add the avocado, and enjoy!

SUMMER COOLING KITCHARI

You can enjoy this Pitta kitchari without overheating.
Just leave out the heating spices like black mustard seeds
and hing, and add some cooling elements like cilantro and
coconut.

SERVES 4

1/2 cup split yellow mung beans (moong dal)
1/2 cup uncooked white basmati rice
1 (1-inch) piece fresh ginger, peeled and grated or minced
1 cup chopped vegetables (one or two types; see Notes, page 173)
1 to 2 teaspoons sea salt (see Notes, page 173)
1 teaspoon ghee, for serving (optional)
Splash of Bragg Liquid Aminos, for serving (optional)
1 small handful of cilantro, chopped, for garnish (optional)
1 to 2 tablespoons unsweetened shredded coconut, for garnish
  (optional)

FOR THE VAGAR (OIL-SPICE MIX)

2 tablespoons ghee
1 teaspoon ground turmeric
1/2 teaspoon cumin seeds
1/2 teaspoon ground coriander
1/2 teaspoon fennel seeds

Rinse the beans and rice together until the water runs clear. You can let the rice and beans soak while you prepare the rest of the recipe.

Make the oil/spice mix (vagar): Turn on your exhaust fan over the stove, as the scent of the spices will be strong. In an 4- or 6-quart soup pot, melt the ghee over medium-high heat. Add the turmeric, cumin, coriander, and fennel and cook until aromatic, about 1 minute. Spices burn quickly, so make sure the vagar dœsn't begin to smoke!

Stir in the ginger. Drain the beans and rice. Add them to the pot and stir to coat with the vagar, then cook, stirring occasionally, for 45 seconds to 1 minute. Add 4 to 6 cups water (see Notes below) and stir. Stir in the vegetables. Cover and bring to a boil over medium-high heat, then reduce the heat to maintain a simmer and cook until all the water has been absorbed, about 15 minutes, or until the kitchari is the consistency you prefer. Toward the end of the cooking time, season with the salt. Remove from the heat.

Place your portion in a large bowl. If desired, top with the ghee and liquid aminos and garnish with the cilantro and coconut. Store leftovers in an air-tight container in the refrigerator for up to 24 hours. To reheat, add some water to the uneaten portions in the pot and cook over medium heat for a few minutes. (Never freeze or reheat in the microwave.)

NOTES: *Ideal vegetable choices for this dish include burdock root, zucchini, green beans, asparagus, carrots, and celery.*

It is important to use sea salt for the extra moisture provided. Do not use Himalayan salt in this recipe.

Use less water for a stewlike consistency or more water for a soupier consistency.

APPENDIX C

Additional Resources

SUPPLEMENTS, TEAS, HERBS, AND ESSENTIAL OILS

24 Mantra Organic, organic herbs, spices, rice, and beans from India: www.24mantra.com

Banyan Botanicals, supplements: www.banyanbotanicals.com

Floracopeia, authentic essential oils: www.floracopeia.com

vpk by Maharshi Ayurveda, supplements: www.mapi.com

Mountain Rose Herbs: www.mountainroseherbs.com

Organic India, teas, spices: www.organicindia.com

Pure Indian Foods, ghee, spices: www.pureindianfoods.com

Pukka Herbs, herbs, teas: www.pukkaherbs.com

WEBSITES AND NEWSLETTERS

These websites and their newsletters will keep your practice rich and vibrant. The teachers and practitioners here have created innovative and enticing ways of incorporating Ayurvedic and Vedic practices into your life.

Amadea Morningstar: https://amadeamorningstar.net/

Laura Plumb: https://lauraplumb.com/

Kate O'Donnell: http://www.kateodonnell.yoga/

John Douillard: https://lifespa.com/

Maharishi Ayurveda: https://www.mapi.com/

Pleasance Silicki: https://lilomm.com/

Claire Ragozzino: https://vidyaliving.com/

Jaisri Lambert: https://www.ayurveda-seminars.com/

Melanie Phillips: https://madhurimethod.com/

Heather Grzych: https://www.heathergrzych.com/

Sandeep and Nalini Agarwal: https://www.pureindianfoods.com/

Banyan Botanicals: https://www.banyanbotanicals.com/

Dr. Robert Svoboda: http://www.drsvoboda.com/

And . . .

Susan Weis-Bohlen: https://www.breatheayurveda.com/

SCHOOLS AND PROGRAMS IN THE UNITED STATES

Alandi Ayurveda Gurukula: www.alandiashram.org/study-ayurveda

The Ayurvedic Institute: www.ayurveda.com

Bastyr University: www.bastyr.edu

California College of Ayurveda: www.ayurvedacollege.com

Kerala Ayurveda University: www.keralaayurveda.us

Maharishi International University: www.miu.edu

Mount Madonna Institute College of Ayurveda:
www.mountmadonnainstitute.org/college-of-ayurveda

NAMA (National Ayurvedic Medical Association) Recognized pro-
grams: www.ayurvedanama.org/educational-program-listings

Southern California University of Health Sciences: www.scuhs.edu

NOTES

CHAPTER 1: THE ROOTS AND RHYTHMS OF AYURVEDA

1. Hippocrates, *Hippocratic Writings*, ed. G. E. R. Lloyd, trans. John Chadwick (Harmondsworth, UK: Penguin, 1987).

2. "Dosha," *Charak Samhita*, n.d., http://www.carakasamhitaonline .com/mediawiki-1.32.1/index.php?title=Dosha.

3. Maya Tiwari, *Ayurveda Secrets of Healing: The Complete Ayurvedic Guide to Healing Through Pancha Karma Seasonal Therapies, Diet, Herbal Remedies, and Memory* (Delhi, India: Motilal Banarsidass, 2007).

4. Robert Svoboda, *Ayurveda: Life, Health, and Longevity* (Albuquerque, NM: Ayurvedic Press, 2004).

5. Jayesh Thakkar, S. Chaudhari, and Prasanta K. Sarkar, "Ritucharya: Answer to the Lifestyle Disorders," *AYU (An International Quarterly Journal of Research in Ayurveda)* 32, no. 4 (2011): 466, https://doi .org/10.4103/0974-8520.96117.

6. Paige Leigh Reist, "The Basics of Ritucharya: Ayurveda's Secrets of Seasonal Eating," The Art of Living, July 29, 2019, https://www.artof living.org/us-en/the-basics-of-ritucharya-ayurveda-secrets-of-sea sonal-eating.

7. Thakkar et al., "Ritucharya."

8. Richard Smith, ed., "'Let Food Be Thy Medicine . . . ,'" *BMJ* 328, no. 7433 (January 24, 2004), https://doi.org/10.1136/bmj.328.7433.0-g.

9. Fred P. Hochberg, *Trade Is Not a Four-Letter Word: How Six Everyday Products Make the Case for Trade* (New York: Avid Reader Press, 2020).

10. Samuel A. Smits et al., "Seasonal Cycling in the Gut Microbiome of the Hadza Hunter-Gatherers of Tanzania," *Science* 357, no. 6353 (2017): 802–6, https://doi.org/10.1126/science.aan4834.

11. "Hadza People," Wikipedia, n.d., https://en.wikipedia.org/wiki/Hadza _people.

12. Jessica Stoller-Conrad, "Microbes Help Produce Serotonin in Gut," California Institute of Technology, April 9, 2015, https://www.caltech .edu/about/news/microbes-help-produce-serotonin-gut-46495.

13. S. M. O'Mahony et al., "Serotonin, Tryptophan Metabolism and the Brain-Gut-Microbiome Axis," *Behavioural Brain Research* 277 (2015): 32–48, https://doi.org/10.1016/j.bbr.2014.07.027.

14. John Douillard, "Lectins + The Plant Paradox: Dr. John's Perspective," John Douillard's LifeSpa," August 1, 2019, https://lifespa.com/lectins -plant-paradox/.

15. Smits et al., "Seasonal Cycling in the Gut Microbiome of the Hadza Hunter-Gatherers of Tanzania."

CHAPTER 2: THE DOSHAS: YOUR UNIQUE COMBINATION OF THE ELEMENTS

1. "Dosha," *Charak Samhita*.

2. Smits et al., "Seasonal Cycling in the Gut Microbiome of the Hadza Hunter-Gatherers of Tanzania."

3. "Your Baby's Dosha," Newborn Mothers, n.d., https://newbornmoth ers.com/blog/your-babys-dosha.

CHAPTER 3: VATA SEASON (WINTER)

1. Dana Cohen, MD, and Gina Bria, *Quench: Beat Fatigue, Drop Weight, and Heal Your Body Through the New Science of Optimum Hydration* (New York: Hachette Books, 2018).

2. "Alternate Nostril Breathing Technique (Nadi Shodhan Pranayama)," The Art of Living, n.d., https://www.artofliving.org/us-en/yoga /breathing-techniques/alternate-nostril-breathing-nadi-shodhan.

3. Harpreet Gujral, DNP, FNP-BC, "Aromatherapy: Do Essential Oils Really Work?," Johns Hopkins Medicine, n.d., https://www.hopkins medicine.org/health/wellness-and-prevention/aromatherapy-do -essential-oils-really-work.

4. Jennifer Lane, "Thieves Oil Recipe—DIY Essential Oil Blend for Protection," Loving Essential Oils, n.d., https://www.lovingessentialoils .com/blogs/diy-recipes/thieves-oil-recipe.

5. "How Do Essential Oils Work?," Taking Charge of Your Health & Wellbeing, Earl E. Bakken Center for Spirituality & Healing, University of Minnesota, https://www.takingcharge.csh.umn.edu/explore -healing-practices/aromatherapy/how-do-essential-oils-work.

6. National Cancer Institute, "Vitamin D and Cancer Prevention," National Institutes of Health, October 21, 2013, https://www.cancer.gov /about-cancer/causes-prevention/risk/diet/vitamin-d-fact-sheet.

7. Jen Murphy, "Finding the Best Time to Exercise," *Wall Street Journal*, June 22, 2015, https://www.wsj.com/articles/finding-the-best-time -to-do-yoga-1434987537. John Douillard, "The Best Workout for Your Body Type," John Douillard's LifeSpa, January 20, 2018, https:// lifespa.com/ayurvedic-fitness-and-body-types/.

8. Deepak Chopra, "Seduction of Spirit" (lecture, Austin, TX, 2009).

CHAPTER 4: KAPHA SEASON (SPRING)

1. John Douillard, "Spring Diet Tips: Ayurvedic Calorie Restriction," John Douillard's LifeSpa, April 18, 2020, https://lifespa.com/spring -calories/.

2. Zoltan Ungvari et al., "Mechanisms Underlying Caloric Restriction and Lifespan Regulation," *Circulation Research* 102, no. 5 (2008): 519– 28, https://doi.org/10.1161/circresaha.107.168369.

3. Bharat B. Aggarwal, PhD, and Debora Yost, *Healing Spices: How to Use 50 Everyday and Exotic Spices to Boost Health and Beat Disease* (New York: Sterling Publishing Co., 2011).

4. Ayman M. Mahmoud et al., "Beneficial Effects of Citrus Flavo- noids on Cardiovascular and Metabolic Health," *Oxidative Medi- cine and Cellular Longevity* 2019 (March 2019): 1–19, https://doi.org /10.1155/2019/5484138.

5. Debra Kamin, "It's in the Weeds: Herbicide Linked to Human Liver Disease," UC San Diego Health, May 14, 2019, https://health.ucsd .edu/news/releases/Pages/2019-05-14-herbicide-linked-to-human -liver-disease.aspx.

6. Gaétan Chevalier et al., "Earthing: Health Implications of Recon- necting the Human Body to the Earth's Surface Electrons," *Jour- nal of Environmental and Public Health* 2012 (2012): 1–8, https://doi .org/10.1155/2012/291541.

7. Barbara Ann Brennan, *Hands of Light: A Guide to Healing through the Human Energy Field: A New Paradigm for the Human Being in Health, Relationship, and Disease* (Toronto: Bantam Books, 1993).

8. Allyson L. Byrd, Yasmine Belkaid, and Julia A. Segre, "The Human Skin Microbiome," *Nature Reviews Microbiology* 16 (2018): 143–55, https://doi.org/10.1038/nrmicro.2017.157.

CHAPTER 5: PITTA SEASON (SUMMER)

1. Sebastian Pole, *Ayurvedic Medicine: The Principles of Traditional Practice* (London: Singing Dragon, 2013).

2. Jennifer Sass, "ATSDR Report Confirms Glyphosate Cancer Risks," NRDC, April 11, 2019, https://www.nrdc.org/experts/jennifer-sass /atsdr-report-confirms-glyphosate-cancer-risks.

3. Emily Dixon, "Common Weed Killer Glyphosate Increases Cancer Risk by 41%, Study Says," CNN, February 15, 2019, https://www.cnn .com/2019/02/14/health/us-glyphosate-cancer-study-scli-intl/index .html.

4. Usha Lad and Vasant Lad, *Ayurvedic Cooking for Self-Healing* (Albuquerque, NM: Ayurvedic Press, 1997).

5. National Cancer Institute, "Acrylamide and Cancer Risk," National Institutes of Health, n.d., https://www.cancer.gov/about-cancer /causes-prevention/risk/diet/acrylamide-fact-sheet.

6. Dana Cohen, MD, and Gina Bria, *Quench.*

7. "Blue Light Insomnia," SomniLight Light Therapy.

8. Kimberly Burkhart and James R. Phelps, "Amber Lenses to Block Blue Light and Improve Sleep: A Randomized Trial," *Chronobiology International* 26, no. 8 (2009): 1602–12, https://doi.org/10 .3109/07420520903523719.

9. Deepak Chopra, "Seduction of Spirit."

10. Junling Gao et al., "The Neurophysiological Correlates of Religious Chanting," *Scientific Reports* 9, 4262 (2019). https://doi.org/10.1038 /s41598-019-40200-w.

11. Venugopal R. Damerla, MD ABoIM, et al., "Novice Meditators of an Easily Learnable Audible Mantram Sound Self-Induce an Increase in Vagal Tone During Short-Term Practice: A Preliminary Study,"

IMCJ: Integrated Medicine: A Clinician's Journal 17, no. 5 (2018): 20–28, https://www.ncbi.nlm.nih.gov/pmc/articles/PMC6469452/.

12. James Nestor, *Breath: The New Science of a Lost Art*. (New York: Riverhead Books, 2020.)

13. Gavin Van De Walle, MS, RD, "5 Ways Nitric Oxide Supplements Boost Your Health and Performance," Healthline, March 25, 2018, https://www.healthline.com/nutrition/nitric-oxide-supplements.

14. John Douillard, *Body, Mind, and Sport: The Mind-Body Guide to Lifelong Health, Fitness, and Your Personal Best* (New York: Three Rivers Press, 2001).

15. Emily Cronkleton, "7 Ways to Use Calendula Oil for Your Skin," Healthline, June 4, 2018, https://www.healthline.com/health/calendula-oil.

16. "How-To Make Homemade Essential Oil Insect Repellent Spray: Tasty Yummies Natural Health," Tasty Yummies, n.d., https://tasty-yummies.com/homemade-essential-oil-insect-repellent-spray/.

17. Mohammad Hossein Boskabady et al., "Pharmacological Effects of *Rosa Damascena*," *Iranian Journal of Basic Medical Sciences* 14, no. 4 (2011): 295–307.

18. Tapanee Hongratanaworakit, "Relaxing Effect of Rose Oil on Humans," *Natural Product Communications* 4, no. 2 (2009): 291–6.

19. "Copper Stills," Copperstills, n.d., https://copperstills.com/.

20. Jade Shutes "Distilling Your Own Hydrosols," The School for Aromatic Studies, n.d., https://aromaticstudies.com/distilling-your-own-hydrosols/.

ACKNOWLEDGMENTS

This book came together as a pandemic swept across the globe. If ever there was a time to boost the immune system and practice self-care rituals, this was it. The premise of this book took on a whole new meaning during COVID-19—a very powerful, timely, and important message about how to heal yourself, stay healthy, and how to move safely and mindfully in the world.

Some of this book was written in beautiful Bozeman, Montana, which influenced me deeply with the presence of family and the incredible landscape of mountains and streams. Most of it, though, was written in Baltimore, where I was born and raised—still surrounded by beauty but of a different sort than Bozeman. Baltimore is where the seasons come on strong: drenching rains, intense heat, vibrant fall colors, and bone chilling winters. What better place to write about the seasons?

Shifting landscapes enriched my writing, as did the experiences of my clients, students, and community. I want to deeply thank all those people who have opened up and trusted me to let the knowledge of Ayurveda flow from my teachers through to them. I am simply amazed at how many people have healed themselves, their families, and even communities through these practices.

Those teachers include people I have met and those I have not, but whose presence in the world has enriched me. Amadea Morningstar was one of my first teachers, and she not only taught me the art of Ayurvedic cooking, she taught me about being true to myself and how to let the wisdom of the ancients to be expressed in my own, unique individual way. Her encouragement and love through the years has probably formed my personal and professional practice more than any other teacher—or friend.

Others who have greatly influenced me over the years include Dr. Deepak Chopra, Dr. David Simon, Wayne Dyer, Philip Goldberg, Marianne Williamson, davidji, Dr. Robert Svoboda, Dr. John Douillard, Dr. Amit Goswami, Dr. Larry Dossey, Esther Hicks, Don Miguel Ruiz, Eckhart Tolle, Eknath Easwaran, Jon Kabat-Zinn, Thich Nhat Hahn, Pema Chodron, Sharon Salzberg, Cyndi Dale, Dr. Vasant Lad, Dr. Ramkumar Kuty, and Yogananda. Eternal gratitude to Swami Vivekananda for bringing the Vedas to the West.

The team at Tiller are spectacular. My editor, Hannah Robinson, taught me a master class in how to get a whirlwind of thoughts together on the page! I thank you so much, Hannah, for your patience and guidance. You are wise beyond your years, lucky girl! And lucky me.

My agent, Marilyn Allen, from Allen O'Shea Literary Agency worked diligently on getting this book into the right hands. I thank you so much and look forward to more to come.

None of this would have come about if not for my friend Tim Hepp, from my bookstore days. Thank you Tim for your enthusiasm and belief in me!

Basically, I am thrilled to be a "real" writer as I enter the sixth decade of my life and all these people have made it possible. I hope to continue to build the team and publish books that offer practices of hope, love, and happiness to all.

Part of that team is Atwater's Traditional Food Café—not one, but two locations where I find inspiration and a place to write outside of home. Your almond milk lattes powered me through much of this book.

And where would one be without friends? My dearest and oldest friend, Dana Pollack Carey, has been there for me since we were twelve years old! Decades and decades of life together, in different countries, cities, and circumstances, Dana and I have always had common ground of love and respect and the best friendship I have ever had. Thank you for being there for me all these years and many more to come.

And lastly to the one who is always first in my heart. My husband, Larry Bohlen. Your support, encouragement, and hugs can get me through just about anything! The trust, love, and home we have created together with our dogs is the most important thing in the world to me. Thank you so much for sharing this life with me.

ABOUT THE AUTHOR

SUSAN WEIS-BOHLEN is a certified teacher of Ayurveda from the Chopra Center and a meditation and cooking teacher. She has been a practicing Ayurvedic consultant since 2008, having studied with many teachers including Dr. Deepak Chopra, Dr. David Simon, Roger Gabriel, Davidji, Amadea Morningstar, Sharon Salzberg, Jack Kornfield, Joseph Goldstein, David Frawley, Dr. Vasant Lad, and many others in the US and India. She is the author of the *Ayurveda Beginner's Guide: Essential Ayurvedic Principles and Practices to Balance and Heal Naturally* and holds a BA in Radio, TV, and Film from the University of Maryland. Susan lives with her husband, Larry, and their three dogs, Ella, Shadow, and Joonie (a rescue from India), in the woods in Reisterstown, Maryland, just outside Baltimore.